Health&Fitness
MAGAZINE

Words Anna Magee
Cover photography Will Ireland
Photography Will Ireland, Danny Bird
Models Halla @ W Athletic, Lara Baumann @ quantumyoga.com
Hair & make-up Claire Portman using Origins and Kerastase
Editor Mary Comber
Sub-editor Eve Boggenpoel
Art editor Claire Punter
Design Holly White

MagBook publisher Dharmesh Mistry
Digitial production manager Nicky Baker
Operations director Robin Ryan
MagBook account manager Katie Wood
Senior MagBook account executive Matt Wakefield
Managing director of advertising Julian Lloyd-Evans
Newstrade director David Barker
Retail & commercial director Martin Belson
Publisher Nicola Bates
Group publisher Russell Blackman
Group managing director Ian Westwood
Chief operating officer Brett Reynolds
Group finance director Ian Leggett
Chief executive James Tye
Chairman Felix Dennis

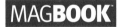

Shape up with Yoga ISBN 1-78106-038-X

To license this product, contact Carlotta Serantoni, +44 (0) 20 7907 6550,
carlotta_serantoni@dennis.co.uk. To syndicate this content, contact
Anj Dosaj-Halai, +44 (0)20 7907 6132, anj_dosaj-halai@dennis.co.uk.

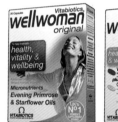
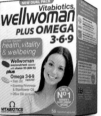
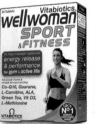
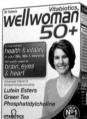
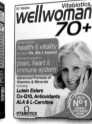
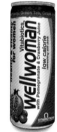

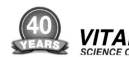
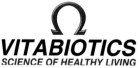

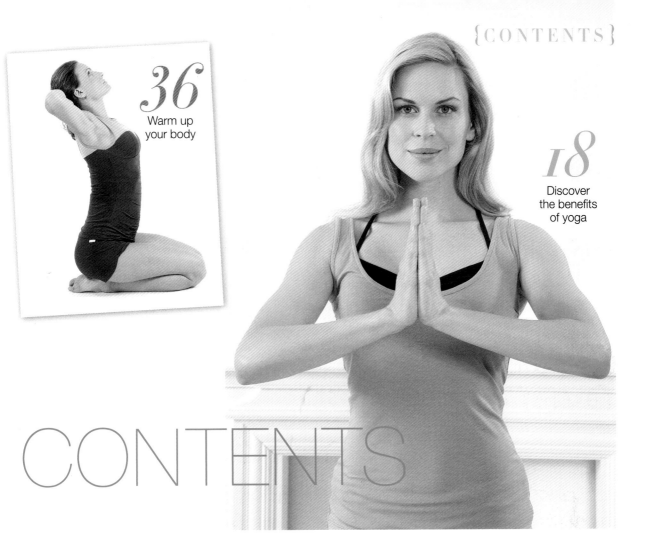

36
Warm up
your body

18
Discover
the benefits
of yoga

CONTENTS

40
Your essential
kit guide

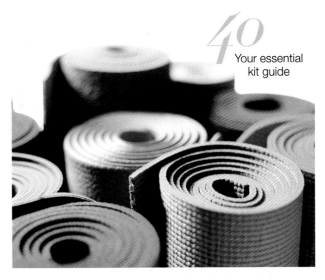

{CONTENTS}

26
Learn the basics

62
Stretch into shape

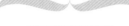

WITH THANKS

With many thanks to Wellicious, the eco-friendly yoga label whose luxury yoga wear and studio feature throughout this book. You can view its latest ranges at wellicious.com. Thanks also to Lara Baumann of Quantum Yoga who models the sun salutations and warm-up moves in this book. Trained by some of the world's greatest yogis, including BKS Iyengar, Lara teaches her method Quantum Yoga across the world and runs Yoga Alliance-certified teacher training courses in the UK. For more information, or to buy her book and DVDs, visit quantumyoga.com.

Wear it
Work it
Love it

Kirsty Gallacher // USA Pro Ambassador

USA PRO

USA PRO

Exclusive to
SPORTS DIRECT.com

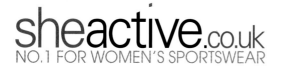
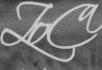

WELCOME

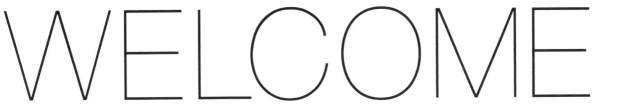

About 14 years ago, I was standing in my dining room having just bought a little book called *Learn Yoga* that lay open on the floor. Clumsily, I reached down to touch my toes. Half way there, I waited for my body to go further, my hands to touch the floor like those of the willowy model in the book. They wouldn't. I couldn't get them past my shins.

Despite my poor old stiff limbs, those few minutes of yogic stretching and breathing made me feel different – shinier, more alert and somehow as though the cobwebs in my head had cleared. That made me want to continue, so I stuck with it.

In time, the benefits surprised me. Yoga toned and lengthened my limbs in ways that years of weight training, aerobics and running never had, and made me feel muscles I didn't know existed. After about six months of consistent four-days-a-week practice, yoga had reshaped my body. But I also slept better and found it easier to stop and pause when I felt stressed or angry.

Today, although I've had many brilliant teachers and become a teacher myself – I can even get my hands flat on the floor! – I'm still thankful to that first yoga book for delivering the clear instructions that gave me my first hint of yoga's rewards, and inspired me to learn more about it.

Yoga's great beauty is that anyone, anywhere, can do it safely and effectively with the right instruction, regardless of how flexible they are. And over time, with practice, anyone can become proficient and discover its astounding benefits.

My mission with this book is to bring you a simple manual to help you learn and safely practise yoga, whatever your level of experience. A little most days is all it takes to help you not only transform your shape and your fitness, but also to feel how yoga's renowned 'buzz' can affect your mood and energy levels.

Most of all, I hope this book inspires you to further explore yoga for yourself, to find your own encouraging teachers and challenging classes, and to practise regularly. It could become one of the most life- and body-changing journeys you ever make.

Namaste

Anna Magee
Author, *Shape up with yoga*

About the author

ANNA MAGEE has been practising yoga for 14 years in various forms, including Iyengar, ashtanga and anusara. In 2010, she qualified as a hatha yoga teacher with London's Triyoga centre, having studied under the inspiring teachers Susannah Hoffmann and Jeff Phoenix, and is a fully accredited British Wheel of Yoga teacher. A multi award-winning journalist specialising in women's health, *Shape up with yoga* is a marriage of two of her greatest loves: yoga and writing. Anna is also co-author of *The De-Stress Diet* (Hay House £9.99).

How to use THIS BOOK

This guide offers all you need to practise yoga at home, from step-by-step posture guides to daily sessions tailored to your goals

To get the full benefits of yoga, it's essential that you learn the basics and build a practice from there. This book sets out the fundamental principles of yoga in practical, easy-to-understand photographs and instructions to guide you every step of the way.

Take your time to read through the book, familiarising yourself with the principles and details of the practices. Once you have the foundations, you can follow the sequences at the back of the book to build up your weekly practice. If you're a beginner wanting to get a grounding in yoga, the six-week plan (page 124) shows you how to use the sequences to grow your experience. Alternatively, practise at your own pace by dipping in and out of the postures. Always remember to do a warm-up to help prevent injury, such as part or all of the one on page 37, until your body temperature rises and you feel more open and centred. Plus, make sure you end any yoga session with some relaxation (page 34) – even two minutes is better than nothing at all!

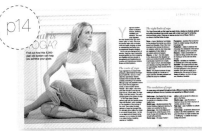

p14

Discover yoga

Learn the history and philosophy of yoga, plus its application in your daily life. Find out what yoga can do for you and how to distinguish your ashtanga from your Iyengar with our simple guide to the styles of yoga – old and new.

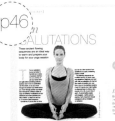

p26

Learn the basics

Discover the fundamentals of yoga and the essentials of breathing, relaxation and meditation. Learn warm-up techniques to help prevent injury and how to use equipment or 'props' to help stabilise and align you, plus essential kit to help get you started.

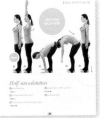

p46

Perfect the postures

We reveal the building blocks of each yoga posture in simple, step-by-step instructions. Alongside each posture, you'll find modifications for your level, experience and ability, plus teaching tips to perfect your alignment safely, to help you get the most from each pose.

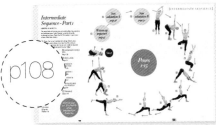

p108

Your daily sessions

Now you can put together everything you've learned with seven, easy-to-follow yoga sequences. There are options to suit all levels – beginners, intermediate and advanced – and goals, whether you want to burn fat, chill out or boost your energy. All the sequences are timed to help you easily fit them into your busy life.

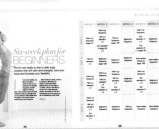

p124

The 6-week plan

This progressive course for beginners incorporates the sequences into a weekly programme designed to give you a grounding in yoga, help you establish your own personal practice at home and progress your technique and fitness.

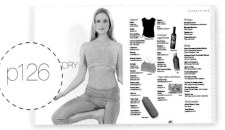

p126

Your yoga directory

Your one-stop address book for all things yoga, including finding a qualified teacher, the best studios, inspiring books and practice websites, plus where to shop for your favourite kit, clothes and props.

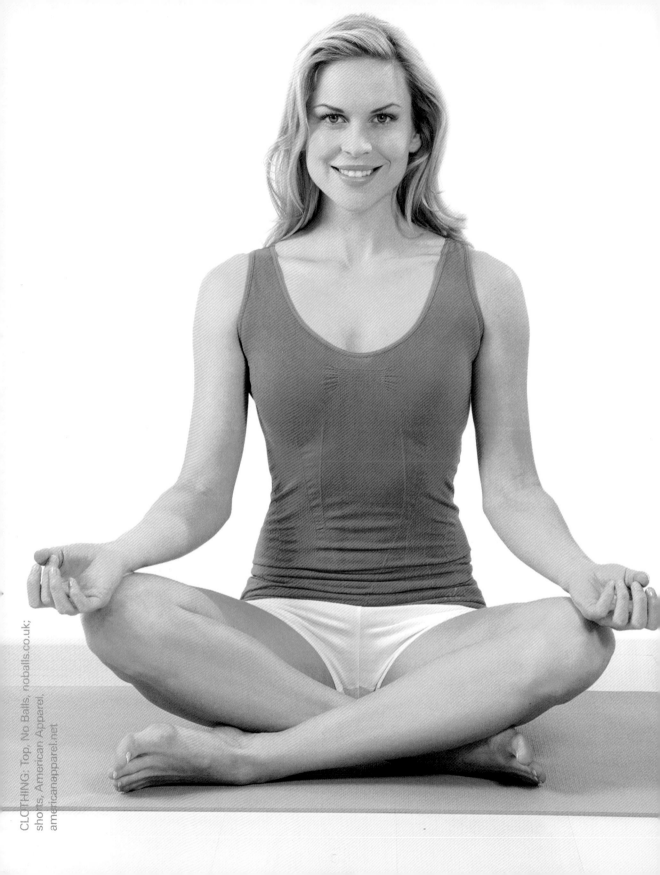

About YOGA

In the West, we often think of yoga as a series of postures that benefit the body by stretching and conditioning it. But yoga is so much more. Most practitioners see it as a complete system of mind, body and spirit fitness that allows us to cope better with the demands of modern life. In this chapter, we explore the history and philosophy of yoga, and how this ancient practice is as relevant today as it was thousands of years ago.

What is YOGA?

Find out how this 5,000-year-old system can help you achieve your goals

Yoga is an ancient system of physical exercise, breathing, meditation and relaxation. The word yoga originated from the Sanskrit word 'yuj' which means 'yoke' or 'union'. Over time, the practice helps unify our bodies, minds and spirits, bringing us closer to understanding and being more compassionate towards ourselves.

But it's not just a feel-good form of exercise. Yoga has many measurable physical benefits too, from increasing your flexibility and bone density to strengthening and lengthening your muscles and improving your posture, fitness and blood pressure.

The roots of yoga

Yoga originated in an ancient Indian philosophy called Vedanta that began around 5,000 BC. Set out in a text called the *Upanishads*, Vedanta maintains that one absolute reality underlies everything in the universe. Although yoga was practised in some form at that time by sages and monks, it was an author named Patanjali – also a sage – who many years later brought us the first real yoga how-to, a book called *The Yoga Sutras*, in the first century. This was a practical guide to the practice of yoga.

In *The Yoga Sutras*, Patanjali defined yoga with the Sanskrit phrase 'citta-vrtti-nirodhah', which translates as 'the cessation of the turnings of the mind'. Even today, the basic definition of yoga has changed little. It's ultimately about stilling the chatter in our minds through focus – be that on our alignment and breath during postures, or on a mantra, the breath or an object during a breathing exercise or meditation.

The eight limbs of yoga

The Yoga Sutras tells us that yoga has eight limbs, relating to physical, spiritual and ethical practices that provide yogis with a total road map for achieving mind and body union. Postures or asanas are just one of those. Here's a run-down of all the limbs of yoga.

Yama – means 'abstinence' and relates to five practices that restrain our actions, speech and thoughts. One of the most important is the concept of ahimsa or non violence, which is why many yogis are vegetarians. It also relates to non-violent actions and speech.

Niyama – or 'law' – this limb relates to five observances that discipline our actions and conduct towards ourselves. A particularly important one is tapas, which means 'to burn', and encourages us to develop a burning enthusiasm for our yoga practice, those we love and for our life's work.

Asana – the physical postures of yoga, intended originally as a small part of yoga's total that ultimately prepared and purified the body for meditation.

Pranayama – exercises that control the breath to unblock energy and purify the body (page 30).

Pratyahara – relates to practices that encourage the withdrawal of the senses which can distract us from our centre.

Dharana – means concentration on an object or thing, and sets the scene for moving on to the next two limbs of yoga.

Dhyana – translates as meditation – an essential part of the yoga equation.

Samadhi – the super-conscious state of awakening in which thoughts are still and total absorption in the moment is possible. Don't get too caught up in achieving this. Any amount of focus – fleeting or lasting – is a form of yoga and, therefore, beneficial.

The evolution of yoga

As yoga grew and spread throughout India, different branches developed, relating to different forms of practice and appealing to different people.

Hatha yoga – the physical form of yoga that has grown fastest in the West. Its purpose is to develop a strong, healthy body.

Bhakti yoga – devotional practices that involve chanting, singing and dancing. Its mission is to worship the Divine.

Jnana yoga – the most intellectual of the yoga forms, which focuses on the study of yoga and controlling the mind, to build self-awareness.

Karma yoga – the yoga of action – selfless work or service for others as a path to the Divine.

Mantra yoga – uses the sense of hearing to focus the mind in the form of mantras, sounds or music.

Raja yoga – uses meditation to cultivate mind control.

Tantra yoga – emphasises pleasure and ecstasy in all of life's experiences – both good and those we might consider bad or challenging – to release the body's energy and power.

Yoga's birth in the West

In the 20th century, a series of revolutionary teachers within India continued to develop different systems in the hatha yoga tradition. For example, in Pune, India, BKS Iyengar created the detailed and structured Iyengar form, and in Mysore, Sri K. Pattabhi Jois created the flowing, dynamic ashtanga style (see page 23).

In the second half of the 20th century – thanks to early Western yoga enthusiasts making pilgrimages to India to learn from the masters, and vice versa – yoga began to flourish in the West. US-born teachers such as David Swenson studied with Sri K. Pattabhi Jois and brought ashtanga yoga to

> 'The sound of "om" is believed to symbolise the vibration of the universe.'

Los Angeles before writing an important practice manual that would lead the way for the system in the West. Then, when Madonna and Gwyneth took it up, there was no stopping ashtanga yoga's popularity.

Westerners began to create their own styles, too – hybrids of what they had learned before. For example, in 1997, John Friend, a US student of Iyengar's, created the now-popular anusara style (page 23).

Yoga's universal appeal is strengthened by the fact that there is no religious dogma that students have to buy into to practise. Yoga is open to all.

Yogic styles and systems continue to change, evolve and re-invent themselves regularly, especially in the West. Still, today's yoga practitioners find that wherever in the world they attend a class and whatever style they choose, there are certain never-changing elements of yoga that are as pure today as they were thousands of years ago. These are focusing, centering and returning to our inner selves and a more peaceful state. They're as relevant – and essential – right now as they ever were.

GLOSSARY

Your beginner's guide to yoga terminology

Asana – a posture or yoga pose.

Kundalini – the positive inner energy or force yogis believe begins at the base of the spine and travels upwards. It's often likened in images to a serpent, and yoga helps awaken it.

Mantra – a short phrase or word (in Sanskrit or any other language, often given to a student by his/her meditation teacher) that is repeated as a focus in meditation or chanted before or after practice.

Namaste – translates as 'the Divine in me recognises the Divine in you'. Used as an everyday greeting in India, it is often said at the end of classes in the West.

Om – written in Sanskrit as 'aum', it's pronounced 'ahh-ohhh-mmmmmm', and chanted on one long exhalation before or after practice or to oneself as a meditation in itself. The sound of 'om' is believed to symbolise the vibrational sound of the universe, and as a therapeutic mantra it's believed its resonance relaxes the mind and body.

Prana – the breath.

Pranayama – therapeutic breathing techniques practised alone or in yoga sessions and classes.

Samadhi – the ultimate state of oneness with all things that ancient (and some modern) yogis aimed to attain.

Sanskrit – the ancient language of the yoga texts, originating in India. In this book, we have provided the Western name of each pose and followed it with the Sanskrit name. According to the yogic texts, Sanskrit words linguistically resonate in ways that are therapeutic for the speaker when they're being said in mantras (see above).

Vinyasa – yoga postures that dynamically flow into one another using the breath.

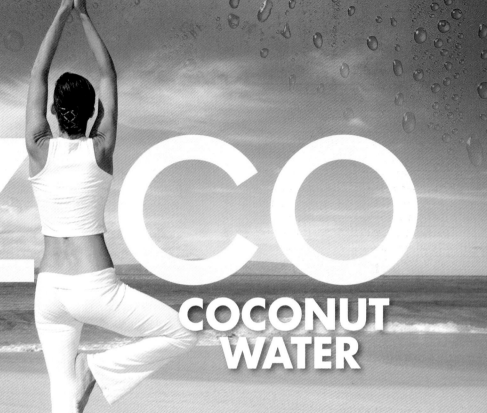

ZICO COCONUT WATER

ZICO: Regain your balance. Renew your day.

ZICO is rich in potassium, the essential electrolyte that helps maintain normal muscle function, and low in calories. With zero fat and no added sugar* it's the ideal way to refresh your day. Now in a re-sealable bottle, ZICO can always be on hand to enjoy the benefits of coconut water throughout the day.

Find ZICO at selected Waitrose & Tesco stores as well as independents across London. For more details visit zico.com/uk.

*Only naturally occurring sugar from the coconuts

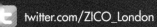 twitter.com/ZICO_London   facebook.com/ZicoUK

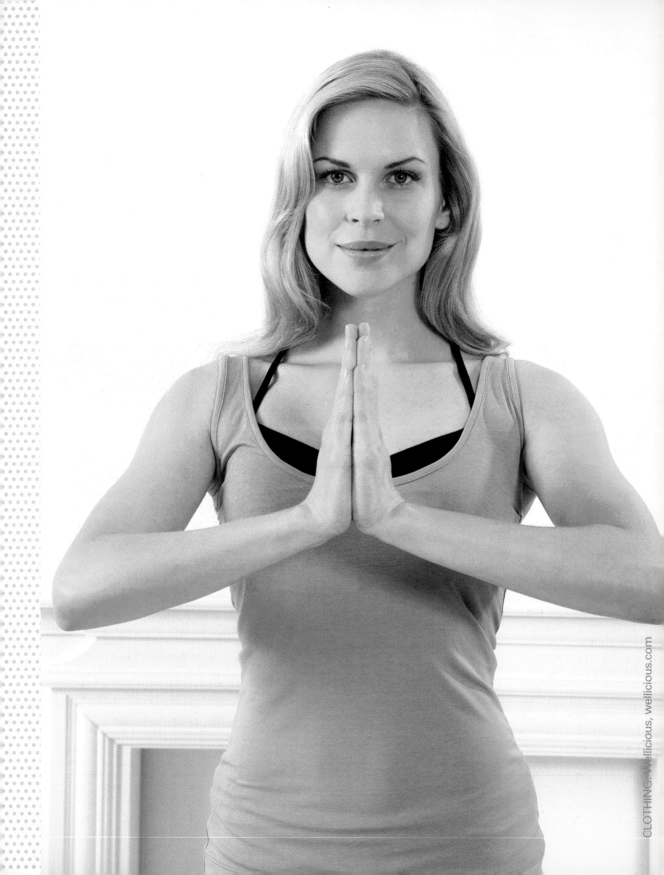

The BENEFITS

Yoga is good for your body and soul, and new research is revealing more and more advantages to following a regular practice

You've probably heard yoga practitioners wax lyrical about the effect of yoga on their minds, bodies and even their attitude to life. Yoga's benefits are now recognised by the scientific community too, with studies showing its benefits on everything from flexibility, bone density and muscle strength to blood pressure and lung capacity.

1) Better flexibility

The mobility and agility of your body depends on the ability of the connective tissues around your joints to expand and contract freely. Age, a sedentary lifestyle, over-exercise, repetitive movements and even stress can all result in your muscles contracting around joints, and this can limit your range of movement, leading to the aches, pains and associated limitations we normally put down to the ageing process.

Yoga lengthens the connective tissues, muscles and ligaments between your joints, so your body's range of movement expands. This, in turn, can reduce the likelihood and severity of injuries both from exercise and in your everyday life – now and in the future.

2) Improved posture

Yoga slowly lengthens your muscles and decreases muscle bulk without sacrificing healthy, lean tissue. Regular yoga practice – especially postures such as lunge twists, bridge, chair and triangle – can also do wonders for your core, the internal 'girdle' made up of your deep abdominal muscles. A strong core is key to staying slim around your middle and helps prevent lower back problems, as core muscles support the skeletal structure in your lower spine. Studies show yoga can lessen back pain over time. A strong core also makes your body appear leaner, longer and toned.

3) Better sex life

One of the best benefits a regular yoga practice brings is to your pelvic floor – the group of muscles that lie under your pelvis and around your sex organs. Postures such as bridge, chair and shoulder stand cause a subtle strengthening of these muscles.

During yoga, some yogis hold an internal lock called mula bandha ('root' and 'lock' in Sanskrit). This involves gently squeezing your pelvic floor muscles between your urethra (where you pee) and anus during each pose, to help strengthen your pelvic floor. Happily, this can also strengthen the muscles that intensify orgasm and prevent the onset of weakened pelvic floor muscles that cause incontinence in later life.

4) Less stress

By encouraging your muscles to relax, and by promoting the stretching of key nerves that link your joints to your mind, yoga can have profoundly de-stressing benefits in just 10 minutes. Practising regularly lowers levels of a stress hormone in the body called cortisol which can lead to weight gain, burn out and exhaustion. Just one hour a week can help reduce stress and anxiety.

A Swedish study found that yoga's benefits were comparable to cognitive behavioural therapy in reducing stress. That's because hatha yoga promotes physical relaxation by decreasing the activity of the sympathetic nervous system and increasing the activity of the parasympathetic nervous system by lowering your heart rate.

5) Optimum health

Yoga has been shown to help decrease blood pressure and alleviate insomnia, headaches and lower back pain. One study found that two classes a week could help improve menstrual cramps and PMS.

Yoga is also a powerful detoxifier. During postures, internal organs are massaged, increasing blood circulation and encouraging detoxification through the lymphatic system. Twists support this internal massaging effect, as the spinal and abdominal rotation cleanses toxins from internal organs much like wringing out a sponge.

6) Better body

Yoga can transform your body's shape. Studies show that regular practice leads to a lower BMI, a reduced waist-to-hip ratio and lower body-fat levels. Research also shows that people who practise yoga regularly are thinner than their non-practising counterparts, have better appetite control and fewer cravings, as well as increased postural stability. What's more, yoga also changes the way you feel towards your body, improving your overall self-image, whatever that waist measurement is!

7) Greater fitness

Practising the more dynamic types of yoga can increase your cardiovascular fitness and help torch those calories. As one posture flows into another and you often jump through postures, you work up a serious sweat. One hour of ashtanga for example, clocks up around 300 calories, while an even tougher power yoga class can burn up to 500 calories and one 90-minute session of Blkram yoga can torch 630 calories.

8) Wider horizons

Think of that point where a muscle stretch feels challenging but can still relax. This is a good form of stress on your body, and yoga can help you become more used to it. This point is what yoga teachers call your 'edge', and finding it, becoming comfortable with it and slowly transcending it is how yoga can help you move through physical and mental limitations. This can also filter into the rest of your life as you become more willing to 'stretch' yourself further.

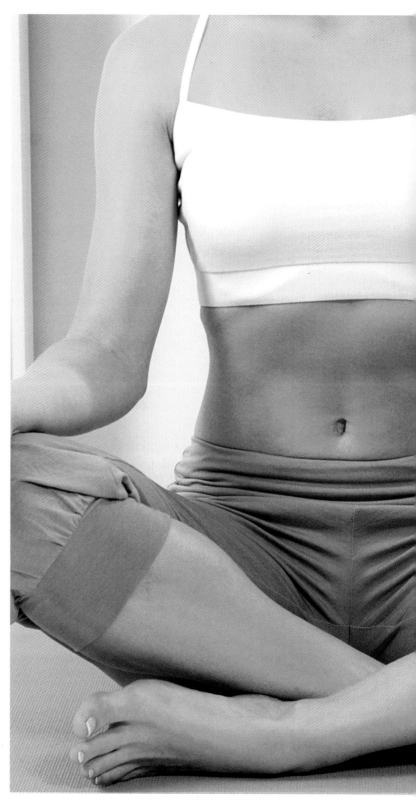

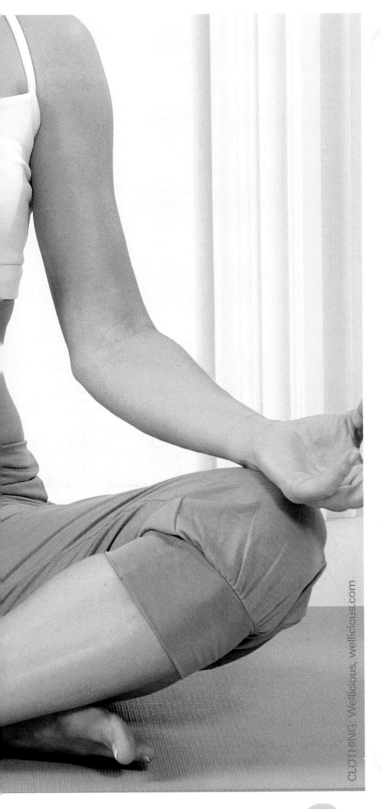

CLOTHING: Wellicious, wellicious.com

YOGA THERAPY

In his ground-breaking book *The Path to Holistic Health*, the pioneer of yoga therapy, BKS Iyengar, outlines sequences and postures that help with specific ailments. 'Yoga is a system of healing based on the premise that your body should be allowed to function as naturally as possible,' he says. 'Practising the recommended asanas will first rejuvenate your body and then tackle the causes of the ailment.' Of course, always seek medical advice for any illness or injury, but here are just a few examples of postures that may accelerate the healing of certain ailments.

Period pain: Reclining cobbler pose (page 81), Hero pose (page 78), Child's pose, supported by lying over a bolster, see modification (page 79)

Headache: One leg bent sitting extension (page 84), Downward-facing dog (page 72), Wide-legged forward bend (page 68)

Lower back ache: Easy cross-legged twist (page 96), Cobbler pose (page 80), Legs up the wall (page 77)

Insomnia: Standing forward bend (page 54), Reclining cobbler pose (page 81), Legs up the wall (page 77)

Constipation: Extended side angle pose (page 66), Triangle (57), Plough (page 75)

Anxiety: Half-moon pose (59), Triangle (57), Seated wide-legged forward bend (page 85)

Exhaustion: Reclining head-to-toe sequence (page 101), Cobbler pose (page 80), Shoulder stand (page 74)

The best
YOGA FOR YOU

Whether you want a slow, static practice or an energetic, flowing workout, there's a style of yoga to suit your goals

From the precision of classic Iyengar classes to the athleticism of ashtanga classes, there are more types, variants and hybrids of yoga to choose from than ever before. Whether you want something to soothe and de-stress or a style that energises and tones, you'll find a method to suit your needs. Ironically, in ayurvedic medicine – the ancient system of healing practised in India – it's believed the type of yoga you're most attracted to is the type you least need. For example, stressed out and high-energy types are often attracted to the structure, routine and challenging poses of ashtanga yoga, but often what their constitution really needs is the deeply relaxing and focusing effects of a gentle and restorative yin yoga practice.

Your starting point should be to learn the basics and fundamentals of yoga (which are similar in most styles) and then try on different types of yoga classes for size. This book will give you a grounding of what constitutes safe and beneficial yoga practice, as you decide which style is best for you.

Look for classes that challenge you while also making you feel relaxed and de-stressed afterwards – without feeling too over-stimulated. Then, pay attention to your how your body looks and feels after a month of regular practice. Your energy should increase, you should feel calmer and begin to see changes to your body shape and feel muscles you haven't felt in a while! If this isn't happening, try something else. Remember, it's perfectly fine to 'mix up' the types of yoga you practice – many yogis do flowing vinyasa classes a few times a week for tone and strength along with a class or two of slow, deeply stretching and enlivening Iyengar practice to stretch their muscles and ground their minds.

HATHA

What is it? Hatha means 'energetic' and it is the basis of all forms of physical yoga that focus on the body. It's primary purpose is to move prana, or energy, through the body using held postures and breathing.

What to expect Classes usually last for 60-90 minutes and include breath awareness, a warm-up to open your joints and muscles, and prepare and open your body, a series of postures held for anything from one to 20 breaths, relaxation, breathing and perhaps some meditation at the end. Postures are usually slow and deep and not as dynamic as styles such as ashtanga or anusara.

Best for Anyone who feels stressed, tired or wound-up. Hatha yoga provides a firm foundation for anyone looking to feel better.

Teacher's tip Opt for a six- to-eight-week beginner's course to teach you the fundamentals of breath and alignment so you can join in classes with confidence.

IYENGAR

What is it? Developed in India by BKS Iyengar, this style is all about correct alignment and the finer details of postures. It utilises props such as blocks, chairs, bolsters and ropes to help release and align your body in postures that are held for six to 20 breaths or even longer. It's challenging but deeply effective.

What to expect There are no sun salutations in this precise system and teachers may give instructions abruptly, so don't take it personally! Some classes focus on a few postures to correct your alignment, which will then affect your practice overall. Expect to feel muscles you didn't know you had.

Best for People who love detail and precision and also want to stretch deeply.

Teacher's tip Make sure your teacher is correctly accredited as this system requires specialist knowledge. Find one at iyengaryoga.org.uk.

ASHTANGA

What is it? Created in 1948 by Sri K. Pattabhi Jois, another of yoga's modern founding fathers, ashtanga involves a series of around 50 postures practised in order. Sometimes referred to as 'power' or 'vinyasa' yoga, it's a dynamic, flowing sequence that creates heat in the body and leaves you feeling sweaty, stretched and invigorated.

What to expect Up to seven rounds of two types of sun salutations make your body hot, then a series of challenging standing, sitting, twisting, inverted and supine postures are held for five breaths each. Classes are rarely less than 90 minutes long and can sometimes run to two hours.

Best for Sporty types, those wanting to get into shape quickly, anyone who likes to sweat and those who thrive on routine and structure.

Teacher's tip People with competitive, type-A personalities are often drawn to ashtanga yoga. Try not to practise from your ego and stay at your own pace. Don't mimic experienced ashtanga yogis in your class – they do astoundingly pretzel-like postures that require strength and skill. Be careful not to run before you can walk in this system.

ANUSARA

What is it? A relatively new style of yoga founded in 1997 by California-based John Friend, anusara has a strong spiritual element to it and is influenced by Iyengar in its focus on correct alignment. Anusara literally means 'flowing with grace' and is an uplifting form of yoga that emphasises flowing, heart-opening postures.

What to expect An energising yoga class experience that works your body deeply, so you will sweat. Classes have an emphasis on bending, rotating and twisting the spine, along with correct alignment. Be prepared also for chanting, breath work, meditation and music (both modern and yogic!) so your mind is fully engaged along with your body.

Best for People wanting a deep workout that is guaranteed to also elevate your mood and introduce you to yogic philosophy in practice.

Teacher's tip A good anusara teacher will make your body feel lean, stretched and opened, and also talk about ways to apply your practice to your everyday life.

SIVANANDA

What is it? Based on the teachings of Swami Sivananda who developed it in the middle of the 20th century, this is a slow, considered form of yoga designed for health and wellness. Its emphasis is on balancing postures with breathing techniques, relaxation and meditation.

What to expect Classes start and end in Corpse pose (Savasana, page 103) which is also practised between the more challenging postures to ensure the body is relaxed after working hard. Breathing practices are done at the start of the class, and only 12 basic postures are then practised, with the aim of opening the energy channels in the body.

'Anusara literally means "flowing with grace" and is an uplifting form of yoga with heart-opening postures.'

Best for Anyone wanting more serenity and a yoga experience that balances the fundamentals of breath, meditation and chanting with a simple posture practice.

Teacher's tip Sivananda is a great choice if you're interested in finding out more about yogic diet and philosophy.

RESTORATIVE

What is it? A series of long-held and supported postures designed to relieve chronic stress and tiredness and restore energy. Postures are usually supported by blankets, blocks or other props.

What to expect Postures are held for up to 15 minutes with the use of props

such as blankets, eye covers, bolsters, blocks and bricks to encourage full support and relaxation. Classes have a warm, comforting atmosphere (sometimes the lights are dimmed and candles lit) but beginners may find them intimidating because of the intense stillness. If you persevere, the rewards will be great.

Best for People who are feeling frazzled and as though they lack 'space' in their daily lives. Anyone suffering from insomnia and stress. Yogis who practise more dynamic styles to help balance out the body.

Teacher's tip Judith Lasater's book *Relax and Renew: Restful Yoga for Stressful Times* is a fantastic reference.

YIN

What is it? Founded by chi kung expert Paulie Zink, yin yoga is a modern yoga style that holds postures still with long, slow breathing to work deeply into connective tissues, promote circulation and help release energy blockages.

What to expect The emphasis is on stretching and opening your muscles, so postures are held for up to five minutes, and you may only get through about 12-15 poses in a 90-minute class! Classes are deeply relaxing and often done with the lights down, so think twice before driving home!

Best for Anyone feeling exhausted or burnt out, with injuries or illnesses and looking to restore their energy.

Teacher's tip Named after the 'yin' of 'yin/yang', this is great as an adjunct to a more dynamic yoga practice or alongside a weight or aerobic training programme to deeply stretch your muscles.

JIVAMUKTI

What is it? Founded in 1984 by artist David Life and former dancer Sharon Gannon, jivamukti is a vigorous form of yoga that emphasises flowing, dynamic moves through postures, coupled with a focus on Indian philosophy.

What to expect A combination of flowing 'vinyasa' postures (with hands-on adjustments for alignment from teachers) along with breathing, meditation, Sanskrit chanting, philosophical discussion and deep relaxation.

Best for Anyone wanting to take a challenging flowing class where they can learn how to apply yogic philosophy to everyday life.

Teacher's tip There is often gorgeous music playing in classes – anything from chanting to a five-piece band!

KUNDALINI

What is it? Uses active and passive postures to awaken 'kundalini' energy, the positive life force that, in yogic philosophy, is believed to be stored at the base of your spine.

What to expect Rapid, repetitive movements that can be quite different from regular postures. Chanting and meditation is included and the teacher may play a gong and sing.

Best for Anyone interested in experiencing the more esoteric and spiritual side of yoga.

Teacher's tip The release of kundalini energy has been practised for centuries. Students can be surprised by the power of this practice and may become emotional during or after a class. Rather than sad, this can be a great release.

....

BIKRAM

What is it? A series of 26 postures and two breathing exercises are done in a standard order in a hot room over the course of 90 minutes. The intense heat warms muscles and joints and encourages increased mobility and flexibility – and sweat, lots of it.

What to expect Classes are usually crowded and mats are often lined up just inches apart during busy times. If you're expecting a quiet, candlelit experience, forget it. Studios are bright and teachers usually blare out instructions through a well-used microphone. Bikram practice can help shape your body and release excess weight, but you need to be consistent and practise around three to five times a week. Make sure you talk to your teacher about any injuries or medical conditions before you begin.

Best for Anyone looking to feel they have really worked out during their yoga practice. Although Bikram yoga can help elevate your mood, philosophy and the spiritual aspects of yoga are rarely mentioned.

Teacher's tip Wear as little as possible! Most people tend to wear shorts and tank tops for their Bikram practice to help them keep cool. Always remember to bring a towel and a large water bottle – you'll need them. As people tend to sweat so profusely, Bikram 'in-house' mats tend to be overused, so you might want to bring your own mat.

'The release of kundalini energy has been practised for centuries, and the class may feel surprisingly powerful.'

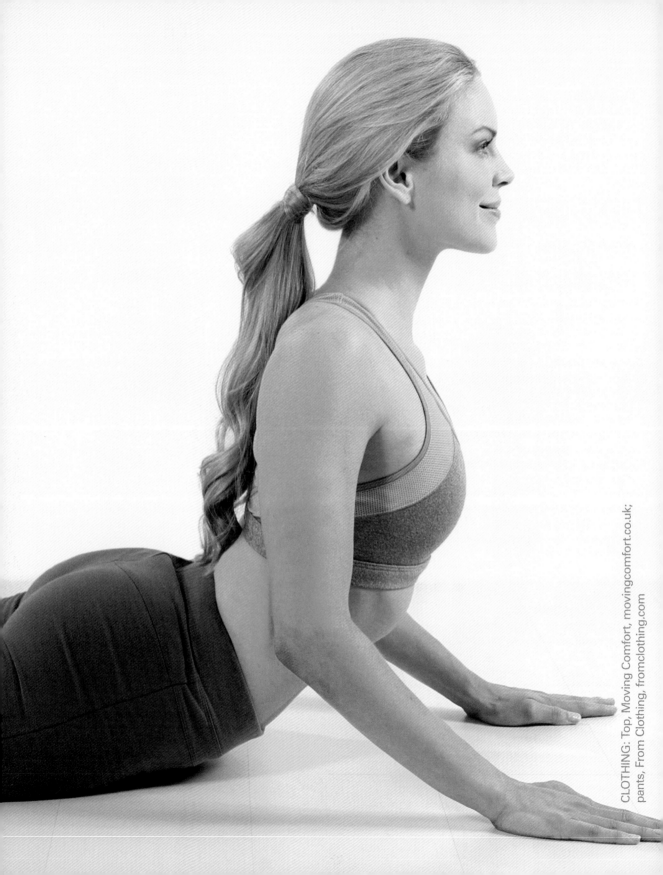

The
BASICS

Now that you've discovered how yoga can transform your mind and body, it's time to get started. This chapter will help you make space for yoga in your life and show you how to prepare your muscles and joints for the postures using correct warm-up techniques. Discover the basic principles of breathing, meditation and relaxation so you can reap the physical and mental rewards of a regular yoga practice.

Make the most of YOUR PRACTICE

Follow these expert tips to get the maximum benefits and enjoyment from your yoga sessions

● Balance your yoga practice by including relaxation, breathing and postures into your workout wherever you can.

● Create a DIY yoga session of your own by including one from each of the following categories: warm-up, standing, balance and sitting postures, forward bends, back bends, twisting postures, supine and restorative postures, followed by a final relaxation.

● If you're practising at home, make the space inviting with anything that appeals to your sense of self – your favourite flowers, relaxing or invigorating aromatherapy oils (citrus and lavender are great), or a photo or symbol that instantly relaxes you.

● Try not to eat for two to three hours before doing yoga so you can move through postures with more lightness and agility (and less indigestion).

● Don't guzzle too much water before yoga – take sips from a bottle throughout the day and afterwards.

● Teachers often sign off by placing their hands in prayer position, bowing their heads and saying the word 'namaste'. This is Sanskrit – the ancient language of yoga originating in India – and roughly translates as 'to be well' or 'the Divine in me recognises the Divine in you'.

● Look for a teacher who inspires you with an understanding of anatomy to complement what you learn in this book. The best ones observe their students as individuals, teaching in a safe, fun environment and challenge them to move deeper into their yoga practice over time.

● If you have any injuries – even old ones – or medical conditions such as high blood pressure, tell your teacher before any yoga class, as this will preclude you from some postures or require you to modify your practice.

● Check with your doctor or physiotherapist about whether beginning a yoga practice is right for you.

● During your period, avoid inverted postures such as Shoulder stand as these can disturb menstrual flow.

● Don't push yourself! Yoga is about allowing your mind and body to open, not forcing it into pretzel-like poses that could cause injury. Yoga's founding fathers talked about the principle of ahimsa or 'non violence', which applies to not being hard on yourself as well as not being hard on others.

● Don't set yourself up for failure by trying to practise for too long. Little and often is best.

● For fast hydration after your yoga session, coconut water (available in most supermarkets and health food stores) provides more natural electrolytes than most sports drinks.

● Fancy playing music during your yoga practice? Deva Premal is a favourite among yoga teachers, especially the album *Dakshina* (£6.32 from iTunes).

● Mix up your practice to suit your energy. Some days you'll feel like a doing a dynamic yoga practice, others you'll be tired and feel as if your body could do with regeneration. During these times, do restorative postures such as Corpse, Legs up the wall and Reclining cobbler, and hold them for longer, focusing on your breath – great if you're lacking sleep.

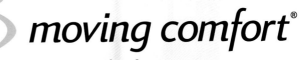

YOGA
breathing

Deepen your yoga practice and boost your health by learning how to breathe correctly during your sessions

An essential part of yoga practice is your breath. Whether it's learning to breathe correctly, moving with your breath through postures or using therapeutic breathing techniques called pranayama to support your mind and body, learning to observe and control your breath in yoga can quickly transform your health and wellbeing.

Most of us don't give much thought to our breath, a process that's even more essential to life than food and water. Consequently, the vast majority of people breathe incorrectly, perhaps too shallow, fast, restricted or habitually uneven. Our breathing is influenced by our moods and lifestyle. During times of stress, we often unwittingly hold our breath and end up

needing to take in occasional big gulps of air. This gives rise to the intermittent loud sighs you often hear in stressed out offices! Better breathing can not only calm and restore your mind and body and help bring you back to the present, it can nourish and detox every single cell and organ in your body – from your digestive system to your skin – from the inside out.

Basic yoga breath
Use these three breathing principles during yoga practice.

1. **Breathe in and out through your nose** – this is considered a cleaner, warmer breath that gives more control and evenness to movement. Obviously, if you have a blocked nose or a cold, breathing through your mouth is okay!

2. **Focus on your breath** – if a posture feels difficult or strained, return your attention to your breath, focus on its texture and try to even out the inhalation and exhalation – both should be approximately the same length – breathing deeply into your diaphragm (see page 32).

3. **Co-ordinate breath with movement** – in yoga, breathing can help movement if you focus on moving with your breath. Throughout this book, posture instructions include breath cues, as will most class teachers. As a general rule of thumb, inhale while opening, lengthening or extending your body, and exhale while deepening, releasing or folding into a posture. Don't fret about getting this right though, by simply focusing on your breath during your practice, it will eventually become second nature.

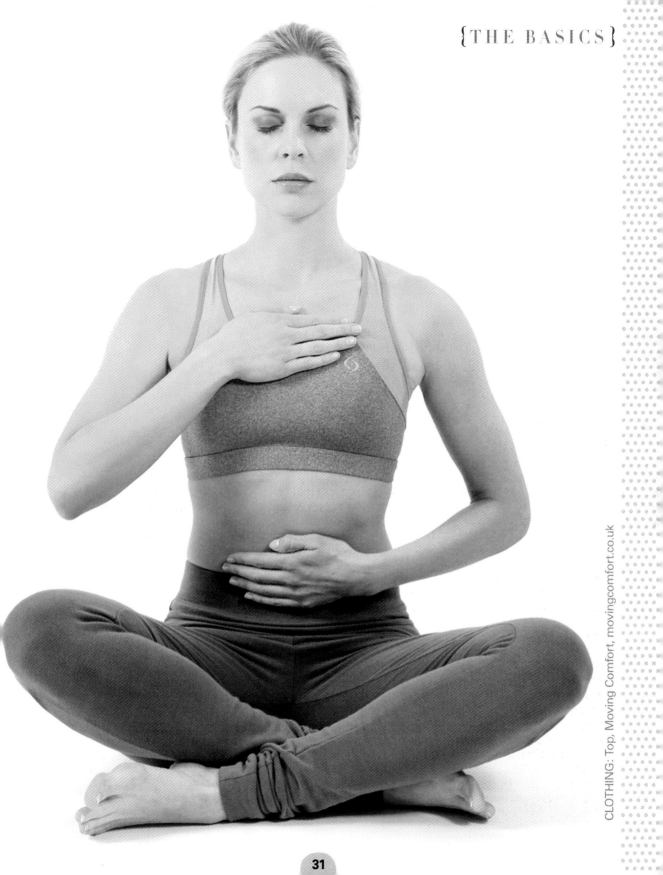

CLOTHING: Top, Moving Comfort, movingcomfort.co.uk

Observing the breath

This is practised at the beginning of yoga sessions to help even out your breath, so you can turn your attention inwards and come into the present before moving through the postures.

How to do it

● Lie down on your mat with your legs out in front of you or – especially if you have lower back pain – with your feet hip-width apart, knees bent and together. Or sit in a comfortable Easy cross-legged position (page 87).
● If you are sitting, lace your hands in a comfortable position on your lap or knees, palms facing up. If you're lying down on the floor, place your hands beside you palms facing up, or on your tummy, palms down.
● Make sure your spine is straight by stacking your shoulders above your hips and lengthening your spine by lifting the crown of your head. Contracting your core slightly will help you hold the pose.
● Close your eyes and feel the movement of your breath through your body. Notice the quality and length of your breathing.
● Observe your breath in this way until you notice it slows down and becomes more even.

● Count the length of each in-breath and each out-breath.
● Notice the small pause after the in-breath and again, after the out-breath.
● Continue observing the passage of your breath.
● Watch your breath gradually deepen. Observe how as you inhale, your diaphragm lifts, expands and broadens your ribcage and your belly opens and fills with air, and how your diaphragm lowers and your ribcage and abdomen contract as you exhale.
● Spend around five to 15 minutes at the beginning of your practice on this exercise.

Breathing exercises

PRANAYAMA

In yoga, controlled breathing practices – known as pranayama – are used for therapeutic benefits. These are powerful practices, so begin with a short session and build up as you become more familiar with them.

VICTORIOUS BREATH
UJJAYI BREATH

Effect Cleansing, calming and invigorating.
When to do it Ujjayi breathing can be done while working on postures or

practised before or after them (before relaxation) for an invigorating effect.

How to do it

● Sit cross-legged or lie down with support, such as a bolster, under your back (above). Broaden your chest and draw in your chin slightly.
● Exhale fully. Inhale through both nostrils and exhale through your mouth, silently making the sound 'ha'. Continue in this way for about three breaths.
● Now close your mouth and continue

silently making the sound of 'ha' as you inhale and exhale. Feel the gentle constriction in the throat this produces and listen to the subtle 'hissing' sound the breath takes on.
● Continue breathing in this way, with your throat constricted but directing your breath deep into your lungs. Feel your chest open and your diaphragm expand sideways as you do so.
● Beginners should only do three to five minutes of this practice, and slowly build up to 10-15 minutes over time.

ALTERNATE NOSTRIL BREATH
NADI SODHANA

Effect Helps combat nerves, panic or confusion. Calms the brain and can also ease sinus congestion. Yogis say nadi sodhana breathing balances the left and right sides of your brain.

When to do it Alternate nostril breath can be done before an event that makes you feel nervous, before bed or anytime you need to feel more centered.

How to do it

● Sit in Easy cross-legged (page 87) or Hero pose (page 78). Use the support of a cushion if that's more confortable.
● Rest your left hand on your left leg and fold the index and middle finger of your right hand inwards to your palm and wrap your thumb around them.

● Draw your chin slightly inwards so your head bows down slightly. Close your eyes.
● Bring your right hand up to your face and use your ring finger to close your left nostril. Exhale through your right nostril.
● Inhale through your right nostril.
● Close your right nostril with your right thumb and release your ring finger from your left nostril.
● Exhale through the your left nostril. Inhale through your left nostril.
● Close your left nostril and exhale through your right nostril. This is one cycle. Inhale again through your right nostril and continue in this way for 10-30 cycles.
● Ensure you are not slouching throughout the practice, and keep your spine long, shoulders relaxed and chest open.

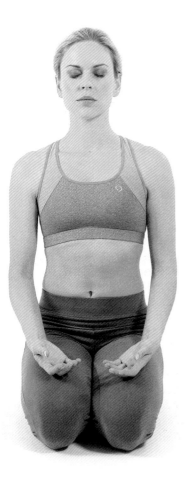

BELLOWS BREATH
KAPALABHATI BREATHING

Effect Known to yogis as the 'cleansing breath', this energises your body in as little as one minute, and also tones your tummy muscles.

When to do it Anytime you need a pick-me-up, such as 4pm most afternoons! Great first thing in the morning but never after eating, during menstruation or if you're pregnant.

How to do it

● Sit in Hero or Easy cross-legged pose and focus for a moment on your breathing.
● Now, close your mouth and, on each exhalation through your nose, simply draw your abdomen inward. Imagine your navel moving upwards and inwards as you exhale. Let the inhale happen naturally.
● Do this a few times and you'll notice your abdomen moving in and out like a bellows.
● Now, speed up the exhalation so you're taking one each second.
● You should be able to hear the exhalation but not the inhalation. This is correct. Do about 15-20 exhalations, rest and start another cycle. Beginners should start with 15 breaths a cycle, and experienced students can do up to 30.

TIP: Focus on drawing your abdomen back, as though you're pulling your navel to your spine on each quick exhalation - about one per second - and don't worry about the inhalation, it will happen naturally.

Relaxation

It's as central to your practice as postures, and will ensure the benefits you experience in class continue throughout the day

We can't escape our need for rest. Part of the rhythm of life, it's natural for all creatures – human or animal – to relax after working hard. Yet in our 24/7 lives, we often delegate restful time to the bottom of our daily priorities.

Yoga acknowledges our need for relaxation both day-to-day and within our yoga practice. That's why yogis often practise active forms of relaxation such as Corpse pose and yogic sleep (see right) anytime they need to feel refreshed and restored.

Why is relaxation so crucial to health? When we do tough physical exercise or mental work, or go through a period under stress, our bodies release hormones such as cortisol and adrenaline to give us the energy and fighting spirit we need to get the job done. But that's only healthy in the short term. If stress hormones hang around in our systems, they can lead to weight gain, sleep problems and stress-related aging. One of the fastest ways to dissipate the stress hormones in your body is to switch on your relaxation response using the yogic practices listed here. If you've ever wondered why you look and feel so much better after yoga, it's because your body has begun repairing itself by switching on your nervous system's renewal processes, helping you recover from stress. So relax, it's compulsory!

Types of relaxation

1 CORSPE POSE SAVASANA

What? A posture in which you lay flat and still on the floor (pictured below), muscles and mind fully relaxed, breathing evenly for two to 20 minutes.

When? Practised before and/or after yoga postures. Some teachers and yoga schools include short Corspe poses, held for about 10 breaths, after challenging poses to help students recover.

Why? Helps your breathing become even and long. Before yoga, it brings your body into the present and away from distractions of the day. After yoga, it helps assimiliate the benefits of practice into your body. It facilliates a long, slow breath that helps nourish muscles and organs so you get the best out of your practice. Many teachers – including myself – consider it the most important posture of any yoga practice.

How? See page 103 for instructions.

2 YOGIC SLEEP YOGA NIDRA

What? A state of conscious deep sleep or relaxation – sometimes called 'sleep with awareness' – usually taken lying down comfortably over 20-45 minutes.

When? Anytime you need to feel more refreshed quickly or before bed to help calm your mind.

Why? It's incredibly rejuvenating if you've not had enough sleep, and research has shown it can also decrease anxiety if practiced regularly.

How? Yoga nidra is best learned in a the context of a class atmosphere or through a recording by an experienced teacher, as it uses guided imagery and body scanning techniques to draw you into a deep wakeful sleep. Guided recordings are available from iTunes – we like those by teachers Robin Barnes and James Jewell.

3 BRIEF RELAXATION POSTURES DURING PRACTICE

A good yoga session combines effort with rest. Particularly for beginners, certain postures can feel challenging deep in your muscles (a good thing!) but too much effort without enough rest and release could leave your body feeling tense, contracted and even more stressed. That's why most teachers will incorporate certain postures into each

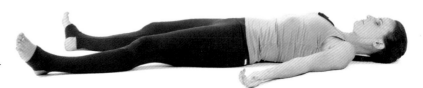

class that serve as relaxation stop-gaps between effortful postures. Here are some of the best:

FORWARD BEND WITH KNEES BENT

This intensely restful pose helps you recover from challenging standing postures such as Warriors I and II and Chair. Done at the beginning of practice, it helps your body become open and relaxed before moving.

CHILD'S POSE

Done with hands by your side or with arms extended and relaxed in front of you, this pose is often practised after difficult poses such as Headstand. It's also often practised near the beginning or end of practice to encourage relaxation and longer, deeper breathing as it makes it easier to breathe deeply to the front, side and back of your body. If any pose feels too challenging, relax in Child's pose until you're ready to resume.

LYING DOWN WITH KNEES BENT

This variation of Corpse pose provides deep relaxation to your lower back, especially after postures such as Bridge (page 93), Wheel (page 95), Plough (page 75) or Shoulder stand (page 74). If your body feels tense during any supine postures, relax in this pose for as many breaths as you need.

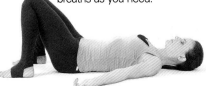

MEDITATION

Known as 'active relaxation' meditation is a central part of yoga. There are many different types of meditation but essentially all of them involve centering and focusing your mind on something. That could be on your breath in breathing meditation, an object such as a candle flame, visualising a beautiful place or simply saying a mantra such as 'om' to yourself.

Why should I meditate? The simple act of sitting and focusing has been proven to enhance mood, boost creativity and increase brain power. It also increases our day-to-day mindfulness, and recent research shows it can help us make better food choices, eat more mindfully and reduce emotional eating.

When should I meditate? Anytime that works for you. Some people find meditating for five minutes each morning works for them, others find 10 minutes at 4pm helps them avoid a vending machine raid by calming the stress that might have them reaching for a chocolate bar.

How should I sit? If you're one of the one per cent of the population who can sit comfortably in Lotus pose, (below) go for it. For the rest of us, an easy cross-legged position with your buttocks supported on a cushion, hero pose or even sitting on a chair work a treat. Your spine should be straight, yet relaxed and open, with your shoulders over

your hips, your chest broad but not stiff and your arms relaxed, hands resting in your lap or on your knees, palms facing up. This allows you to breathe effectively and easily. The main thing is that you feel comfortable yet alert.

But I can't stop my thoughts... Don't worry, nor can anyone. If you're alive, you're thinking! Meditation isn't about reaching some enlightened state of nirvana. Instead, it's about learning to observe and sit with your thoughts and focus on the present moment regardless. Studies show that even people who think that they're not meditating very well are getting the mind-clarifying and calming benefits.

How should I get started? Mindfulness meditation teaches you to observe and let go of thoughts and feelings. It trains you to understand that feelings and thoughts are impermanent and can't hurt you. It has also been proven to help decrease depression, anxiety and insomnia.

Preparing YOUR BODY

*I*magine driving a car without letting the engine warm up or baking a cake without preheating the oven. Okay, so not exactly the end of the world but your results might not be as good as you'd hoped. So too with yoga, warming up the body – even for just a few minutess – is essential to the quality of the postures that follow in your practice and how they affect your body. An adequate warm-up gets you in touch with breath, too, and releases tension. A relaxed body breathes better, and a body that breathes better performs exercise more safely and effectively without unnecessary strain and effort.

From a physiological perspective, warming up is crucial for your muscles and joints. It stimulates blood flow and circulation which helps deliver oxygen and nutrients to cells. This makes more energy available to your muscles for the demanding movements that follow in your yoga practice. Furthermore, a good warm-up stimulates synovial fluid, a thick viscous substance in your joint cavities that provides cushioning and lubrication for joints as they move and helps prevent creakiness and joint pain. After the age of 35, synovial fluid diminishes (one reason old people have a creaky reputation!). The best way to stimulate synovial fluid before yoga is to take key joints through their full range of movements – just what we're about to do.

CLOTHING: Wellicious, wellicious.com

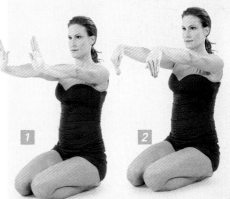

YOGA WARM-UP SEQUENCE

This body prep sequence should take you around five minutes. Follow the instructions below before you begin your yoga sequence so your body is safely warmed and ready for movement. Once you have the hang of the moves, feel free to use any of them anytime you're feeling stiff or tense – such as after commuting, lifting children or sitting for hours at your desk! When they get the hang of them, students often find the moves deliciously relaxing and invigorating even done on their own. Unless otherwise stated, complete 10 cycles of each.

WRIST BENDS

Good for Lubricating your wrist joints (important for yoga but also for carrying shopping and handbags!). Warms forearm muscles.

How-to Sit in any comfortable position on the floor such as Hero or Easy cross-legged pose, arms outstretched. On an inhalation, bend each wrist so the back of your hand moves towards you (1), and, on an exhalation, bend your wrists so your palms are facing you from underneath your wrists (2). This is one cycle. Do five cycles.

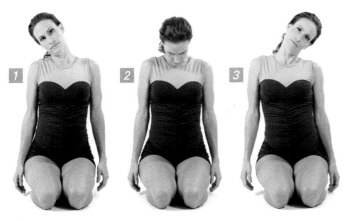

NECK ROLLS

Good for Releasing stiffness, tension and heaviness that accumulate commonly in the neck.

How-to Sit in any comfortable position on the floor such as Hero (page 78) or Easy cross-legged pose (page 87). Keeping your shoulders still, inhale, and bring your right ear as close as possible to your right shoulder (1). Exhale, and draw your chin to your chest (2), inhale, then draw your left ear round close to your left shoulder (3), still keeping your shoulders still. Exhale, and return your head to the starting position. This is one cycle. Complete five cycles in each direction.

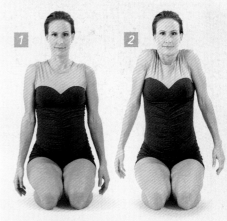

SHOULDER SHRUGS

Good for Releasing any tension held in your shoulders.

How-to Sit in any comfortable position on the floor such as Hero or Easy cross-legged pose (1). Keeping your arms relaxed, inhale and lift your shoulders as close to your ears as you can (2). On an exhalation, release your shoulders down. This is one cycle. Do five cycles.

SAFETY TIP: Never let your head tilt backwards during neck rotations as it strains your neck. If you'd like to stretch your head back, support it by clasping your hands behind your head before you tilt it back.

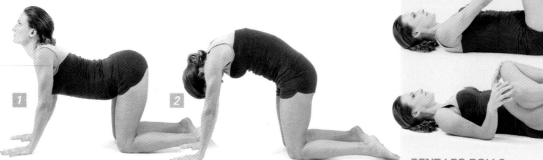

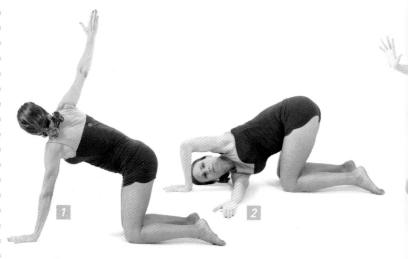

CAT STRETCH

Good for Warming your spine, pelvic area and core muscles.

How-to Start on all fours, hands under shoulders fingers fanning out, knees under hips. Inhale, and gently move your tailbone toward the ceiling, slightly concaving your back (don't drop your belly though, keep your abdominal muscles engaged throughout the move) and draw your shoulders back and down. Look up gently but keep your neck long, don't throw your head back (1). Exhale and tuck your tailbone under, so your pelvis rotates inward toward your chest. Round your back, curving your mid-spine to the ceiling and look down toward your belly (2). This is one cycle. Complete five cycles.

BENT LEG ROLLS

Good for Warming up your hip joints and preparing them for the rotation required in many postures. Great if you sit all day. Encourages your body to relax and release.

How-to Lie on the floor with your legs apart and bent to your chest. Place your hands on your knees and make small, slow circles (1). As your hips warm up, make the circles a little larger (2). Do 10 in each direction.

THREADING THE NEEDLE

Good for Warming your spine for twisting postures, preparing your shoulders and arms, and opening your chest.

How-to Start on all fours, hands under shoulders, knees under hips. Inhale, and lift your right arm up to the ceiling so your shoulder moves with it, and rotate your torso to look up towards it (1). Exhale, and bring your arm down and under your left shoulder, bending your left elbow at a right angle and lowering your hips a little but still keeping them raised a few inches above your calves (2). This is one cycle. Complete five cycles on each side.

OPEN AND CLOSED FISTS

Good for Great for relieving finger tension from typing, texting or writing.

How-to Sit in any comfortable position on the floor such as Hero or Easy cross-legged pose. On an inhalation open your hands as widely as you can, palms down, fingers stretching and fanning out (1). On an exhalation, close your fingers to make a tight fist with your thumb inside (2). This is one cycle.

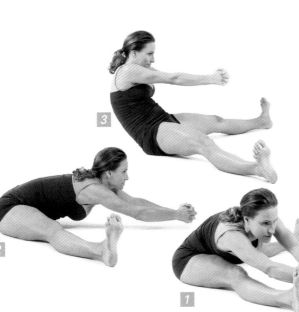

STIRRING THE POT

Good for Opening and warming up your hips, groin, legs and tummy.

How-to Sit on the floor with your legs comfortably apart at right angles. Interlock the fingers of both hands and hold your arms straight out in front of your chest. Inhale, and, keeping your arms straight, tilt your torso towards your right foot (1), and remaining bent forward, continue towards the front (2) and then back towards your left foot. Now, exhale and tilt your torso backwards (3) and round toward to your right, keeping the same arm motion. This is one cycle. Inhale and begin another cycle. Complete at least five cycles in each direction.

TOE SQUEEZES

Good for Preparing your toes and feet for 'rooting' action during standing postures and for decompressing toes that have been squeezed into shoes for long periods.

How-to Sit comfortably with your legs straight out in front of you – or lie down with your legs bent to your chest. Now inhale and as you exhale, bend your toes and squeeze them together, towards the sole of your foot (1). Inhale, release and stretch your toes, separating them as far apart as you can (2). This is one cycle.

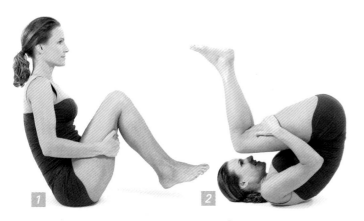

SPINE ROLLS

Good for Massaging your entire spine, hips, pelvis and buttocks. Great first thing in the morning or if you've been sitting at a desk all day.

How-to Sit or lie flat on your back, knees bent to your chest. Hold the backs of the thighs. Keeping your chin close to your chest and abdominals engaged, raise your feet (1) and roll your body forward and back in a rocking motion (2). Your body should gain its own momentum so you feel a massage through your entire spine. Repeat five to 10 times.

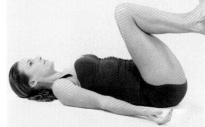

FOOT ROTATIONS

Good for Lubricating your ankle joints and preparing for standing and balance posture. Helps relieve tired or cramping feet.

How-to Lie down with your feet bent to your chest. Now imagine you are drawing big circles in the air with your big toes. Make clockwise circles 10 times and then anti-clockwise circles 10 times.

Your YOGA KIT

Just a few simple pieces of equipment will enhance
your practice and give you the support you need

One of the best things
about yoga is that all
you need is a mat, your
body and a willing mind!
However, certain pieces
of equipment can help.
Moving too far or too quickly into a pose,
can result in unnecessary pain or injury,
ruining your experience of yoga. Whether
it's with a bolster, brick, block or strap,
using equipment can help your body
open at its own pace and lead to better
flexibility. These items can support your
body through modified versions of poses
you might otherwise find challenging,
to ensure safe and correct alignment.

Called yoga 'props', equipment can
also modify postures from active to
passive. For example, after holding an
'active' stretch in say, Cobbler pose (page
80) you can place a bolster, against the
base of your back and release your back
onto it to encourage deep opening in
your chest. In effect, balancing out your
body after the strength-building and
toning action of active poses.

6 OF THE BEST YOGA PROPS

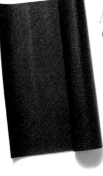

Mat

Called a 'sticky mat', this is specially fabricated to help your feet, hands and other parts of your body avoid slipping when in contact with it. Though prices vary on yoga mats, their basic function is the same so there's no need to spend lots of money on one!

Block

A light rectangular prism made of foam and about one-and-a-half inches thick, a block is great for sitting on to support your back or using as a support for your hands during standing postures, such as Extended side angle pose (page 66), or for the head during Corpse pose (page 103).

Brick

Made of wood traditionally (some modern versions are more lightweight and made of foam), bricks help support your head in forward bends, your back in back bends, and your limbs in all sorts of poses. Improvise with a thick book.

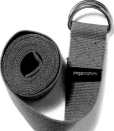

Strap

Excellent for helping you stretch through poses such as forward bends with correct alignment, especially where your hands may not easily reach your feet.

Bolster

Supports your body in supine poses while encouraging it to stretch and relax without any strain. Most have removable cotton covers for washing. You can improvise with a thick, rolled-up blanket.

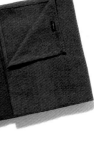

Blanket

Used thinly-folded, blankets can support your back and open your chest in supine and inverted postures. They can also be tightly rolled up to support your neck in some back bends and placed under your knees in relaxation to release your lower back.

All kit available online at yogamatters.com

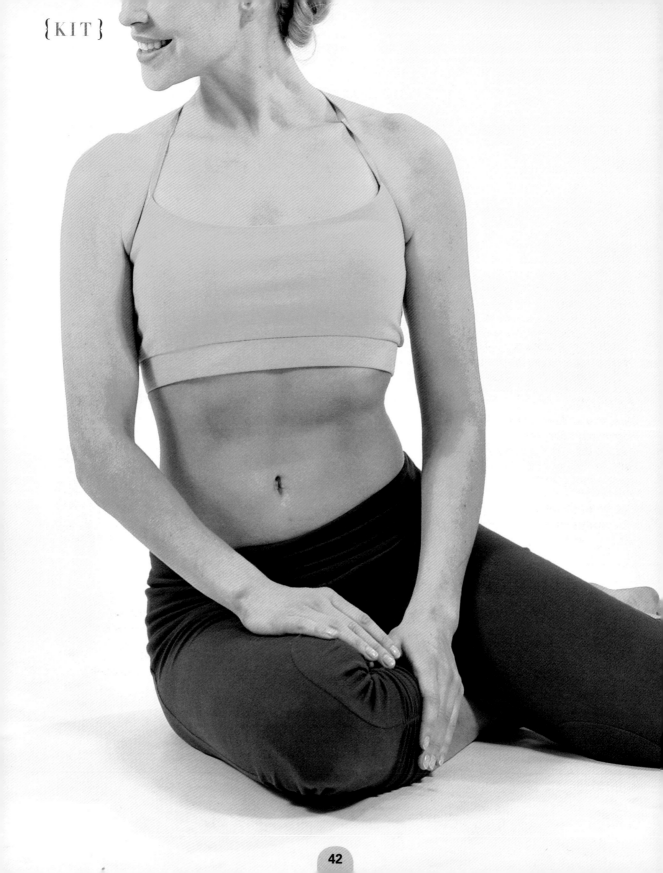

7 YOGA KIT ESSENTIALS

Anyone who has ever been to a yoga class will tell you – it doesn't matter what you wear, as long as you are comfortable. But classical teachers such as BKS Iyengar, one of yoga's modern founding fathers, encourage students to wear clothes that sit snug, but don't constrict the body too much. This helps your body move unencumbered by baggy, hanging fabrics. In a class situation, it means your teacher can observe the small muscular details they need to see to gauge whether you are in a posture safely and beneficially.

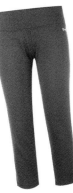

The pants

For agility and ease of movement, look for well-fitting pants cropped either at your shin, knee or thigh. Waistbands that fold over your abs mean pants remain steady and don't ride up or down. More flattering, too! **TRY: USA Pro Three Quarter Leggings; sportsdirect.co.uk/USA-Pro**

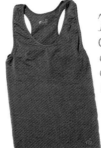

The tank

Choose anything that feels comfortable, though racer or cross-over backs allow for more movement of your upper body without having to worry about falling straps. **TRY: No Balls Seamless Tank with Bra; noballs.co.uk**

The bra

Okay, so you're not running a marathon but support is essential, as postures mean your body makes many different gravity-defying angles, so always wear a sports bra. **TRY: DANS-EZ Minimal Bounce Bra; dans-ez.com**

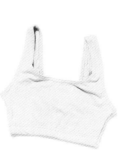

The long-sleeved T-shirt

Your body temperature can fluctuate during yoga practice, so begin with a longer-sleeved T-shirt during cooler weather and strip down to your vest as you warm up. **TRY: Half Moon Yoga Long Sleeved Tee; sweatybetty.co.uk**

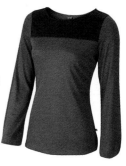

The cover-up

A cosy cover-up or shawl is useful to keep you warm during Corpse pose or meditation – and can also double up as a warm scarf for your trip to class. **TRY: Devi Yoga Shawl; sweatybetty.co.uk, or Asquith Bamboo Scarf; yogabliss.co.uk**

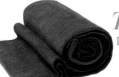

The towel

During dynamic, ashtanga and Bikram sessions you will sweat. Look for a towel made from microfibre fabric for handy packing. **TRY: Manduka Equa Towel; fushi.co.uk**

The mat bag

Invested in your own mat? Portability can be an issue, so a handy mat bag has great compartment action to fit your phone, travel card, water, keys and other essentials. **TRY: Manduka Mat Sack; fushi.co.uk**

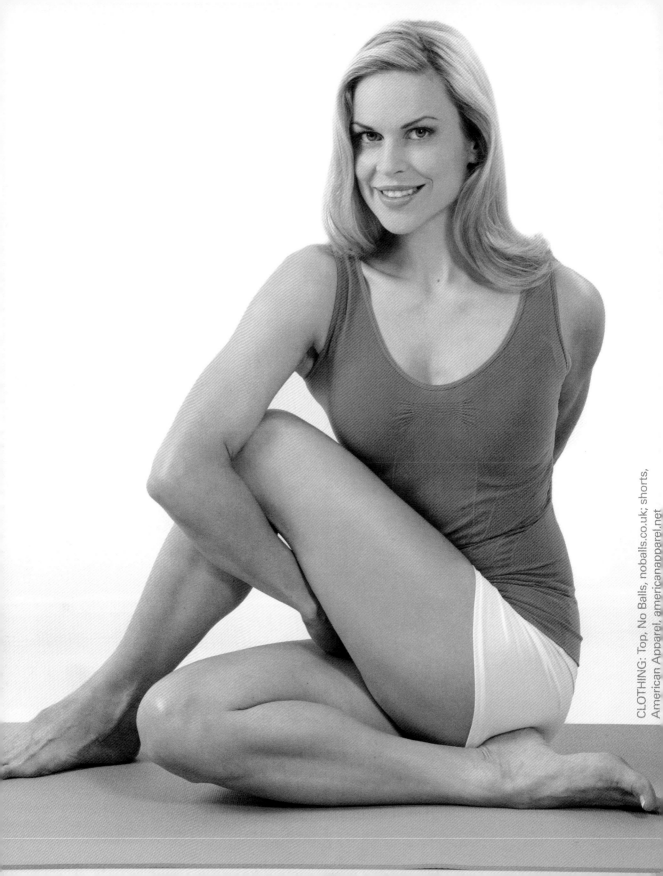

CLOTHING: Top, No Balls, noballs.co.uk; shorts, American Apparel, americanapparel.net

The POSTURES

Welcome to the foundation of your practice, the yoga postures. Here you'll find three types of sun salutation to warm your body before your practice and over 50 yoga postures plus variations for using props. Read carefully through each posture before attempting it. We hope what you learn will deeply stretch, tone and strengthen your muscles, bring calm and clarity to your mind and transform you inside and out.

Sun SALUTATIONS

These ancient flowing sequences are an ideal way to warm and prepare your body for your yoga session

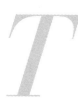he sun salutations (surya namaskar in Sanskrit) are a series of postures that flow into one another, to get your body warm and agile before practising postures (asanas). Each move is coordinated with the breath, so as you move through one posture you inhale and as you move through another you exhale (see instructions). Different styles of yoga use different modifications of sun salutations but all are practised one after another – at least two and up to 12 rounds of each sequence.

Sometimes, if you're short on time,

you can do a few rounds of sun salutations as a quick, awakening practice in itself.

The following sequences are modified versions of classic yogic sun salutations. Beginners can start with Half sun salutations for the first few weeks of practice and, over time, move on to practising versions A and B. If you're at an intermediate or advanced level, try doing a few rounds of A or B, or up to five of each – if you're feeling supple and energetic – before posture practice. Each movement should correspond with an inhalation or exhalation.

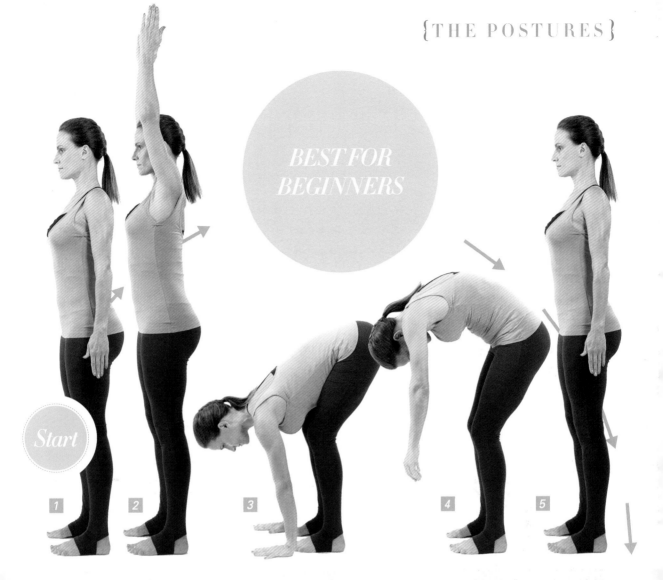

BEST FOR
BEGINNERS

Start

1 2 3 4 5

Half sun salutation

1 MOUNTAIN POSE

Inhale to

2 EXTENDED MOUNTAIN POSE

Exhale to

3 STANDING FORWARD BEND (BENT KNEES)

Inhale and

4 SLOWLY ROLL SPINE BACK UP

Exhale to

5 MOUNTAIN POSE

Sun salutation A

1 MOUNTAIN POSE

Inhale to

2 EXTENDED MOUNTAIN POSE

Exhale down to

3 STANDING FORWARD BEND

Inhale and, keeping your back straight, raise your head and chest to look forward to

4 STANDING FORWARD BEND HEAD FORWARD

Exhale, step your right foot back, inhale and raise your arms to

5 CRESCENT MOON POSE

Exhale, take your hands to the floor and your left foot back to meet your right to

6 DOWNWARD-FACING DOG

Take five deep breaths. Inhale, and bring your right foot forward to

7 CRESCENT MOON POSE

Exhale, hands to the floor and bring your left foot forward to meet your right. Inhale and, keeping your back straight, lift your chest and look forward to

8 STANDING FORWARD BEND HEAD FORWARD

Exhale to

9 STANDING FORWARD BEND

Inhale, slowly roll up to

EXTENDED MOUNTAIN POSE (PIC TWO)

Exhale to

MOUNTAIN POSE (PIC ONE)

Repeat on the opposite side.

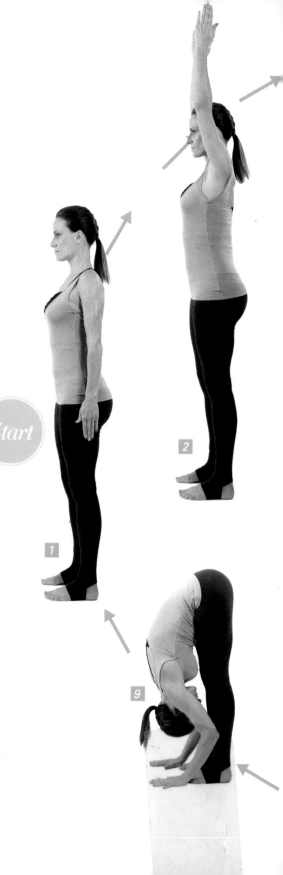

Start

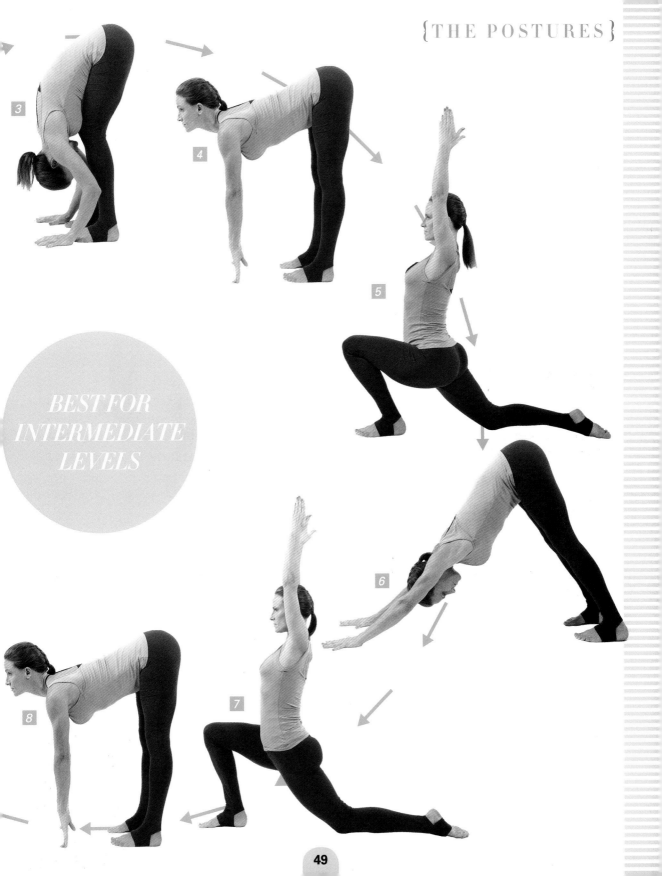

BEST FOR INTERMEDIATE LEVELS

Sun salutation B

1 MOUNTAIN POSE

Inhale to

2 EXTENDED MOUNTAIN POSE

Exhale down to

3 STANDING FORWARD BEND

Inhale and, keeping your back straight, lift your head and chest to look forward to

4 STANDING FORWARD BEND HEAD FORWARD

Exhale, step (intermediate or advanced may jump) your feet back to

5 PLANK

Inhale, lift your hips up to

6 DOWNWARD-FACING DOG

Take five deep breaths, focusing on the alignment of your feet and hands, and on your breath.

7 SLIDING SERPENT

On a long inhalation, bend your knees to touch the mat and, keeping your hips raised, bring your chin to the floor. Draw your body forward, as though you are pushing a golf ball with your chin to the front of the mat until you are laying flat, face down.

8 COBRA

Exhale, press your arms into the mat, lift your body into

9 DOWNWARD-FACING DOG

Inhale, step or jump your feet forward to

10 STANDING FORWARD BEND HEAD FORWARD

Exhale and fold your body forward to

11 STANDING FORWARD BEND

Inhale, roll up and exhale to

MOUNTAIN POSE (PIC ONE)

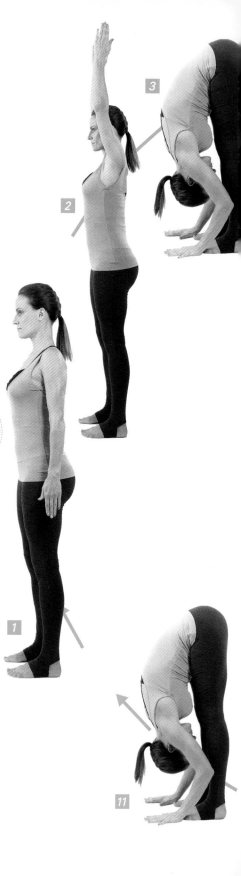

Start

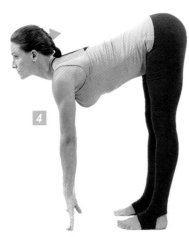

4

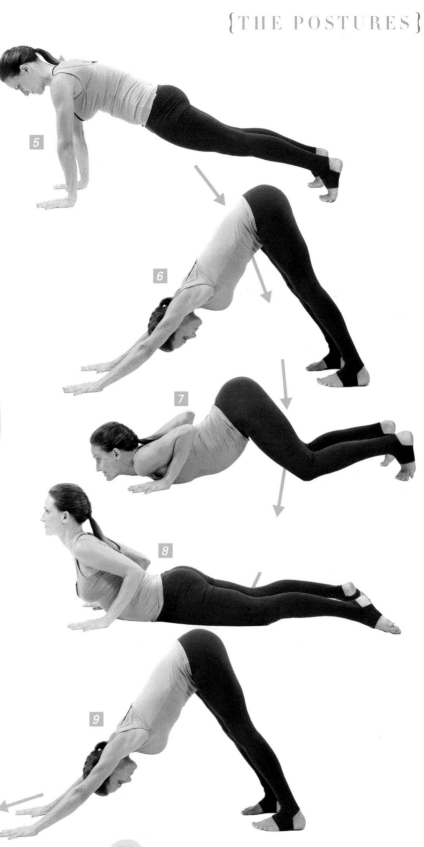

5

6

7

8

9

10

BEST FOR
INTERMEDIATE
& ADVANCED
LEVELS

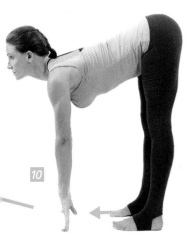

Mountain pose
TADASANA

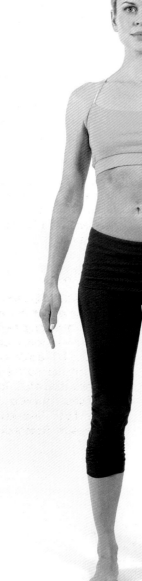

Benefits

MIND – encourages focus and calm.
BODY – improves posture, strengthens your legs.

● Stand with your feet together, ankles behind your toes or (if you have stiff knees or lower back) hip-distance apart, feet parallel.

● Imagine each foot as having four points at each corner, and root your weight down evenly on all four corners of your foot.

● Lift the inner arches of your feet. Press the top of your thigh muscles back towards your thigh bones.

● Lengthen your tailbone to the floor so your spine becomes straight.

● Gently lift the front of your chest.

● Softly extend your arms down by the sides of your legs, fingers pointing down.

● Lengthen the back of your neck and extend the crown of your head upwards.

● Relax your shoulders.

● Take five to 10 breaths.

TIP
Draw your ribs and core gently inwards as you lengthen your spine by extending your tailbone downwards.

Extended mountain pose

URDHVA HASTASANA

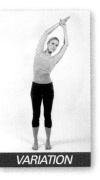

VARIATION

Benefits

MIND – enlivening and energising.
BODY – encourages deeper breathing, stretches your oblique muscles.

● Begin in Mountain pose (facing page) centering your weight on all four corners of your feet, focusing on your breath.

● Turn your palms outward, inhale and lift your arms out to the side and up towards the ceiling, stopping when they're parallel. This is the classic pose.

● Reach up through your hands without compressing your neck and keep your shoulders down. Take deep five breaths.

Variation

On an exhalation, reach both arms over to your left, feeling a stretch in your right side – don't let your torso come forward (this is a side stretch so it's better to move a little to the side than a lot). Take hold of your right wrist with your left hand. Take two to three breaths. Repeat on the other side.

TIP
As you stretch to your left, press your right foot into the floor and vice versa, for a deeper stretch.

Standing forward bend

UTTANASANA

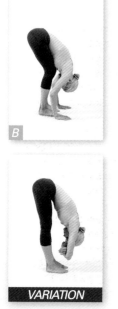

B

VARIATION

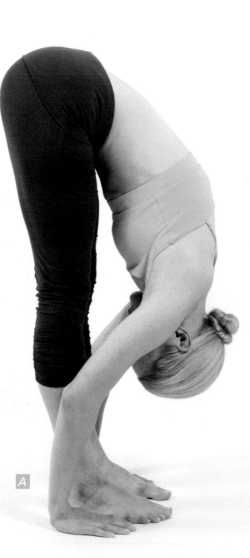

A

Benefits

MIND – deeply relaxing, relieves tiredness.
PHYSICAL – strengthens and stretches your hamstrings, tones your spine.

● From Mountain pose (page 52), inhale and lift your arms up over your head.

● Exhale, bend your knees slightly and fold forward from your hips (not your waist). Relax your upper body toward the floor.

● Place your hands next to your feet (A). If your hands don't easily touch the floor, bend your knees further, ensuring they remain above your feet (B).

● Take five to 10 breaths.

● On an inhalation, slowly roll upwards, uncurling your spine and imagining you're stacking one vertebra over the other until your spine is straight.

Variation

For a super-relaxing tension reliever, fold your arms as you bend over and let your head hang loosely.

Chair
UTKATASANA

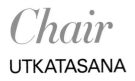

A

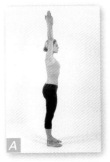

B

Benefits

**MIND – increases clarity and stamina, energises.
BODY – tones your legs and hips, stretches your calves.**

● Stand in Mountain pose (page 52), feet hip-distance apart. Inhale, and lift your arms over your head, palms facing inwards (A).

● As you exhale, bend your knees and lower your hips, as though you are sitting down onto an imaginary chair, until your thighs are almost parallel to the floor (B). Tuck your tailbone under and lengthen your spine.

● Do not let your knees project out over your toes – as you look down you should be able to see your big toes.

● Look straight ahead, relax your shoulders and take five breaths, sinking a little deeper in each exhalation (C) and lengthening your torso on each inhalation.

Variation

To increase inner thigh tone, squeeze a block or thick book between your legs.

C

TIP
Make it dynamic – move with each breath from Mountain pose into Chair, then into forward bend and back to Mountain pose. Repeat five times.

Tree

VRKSASANA

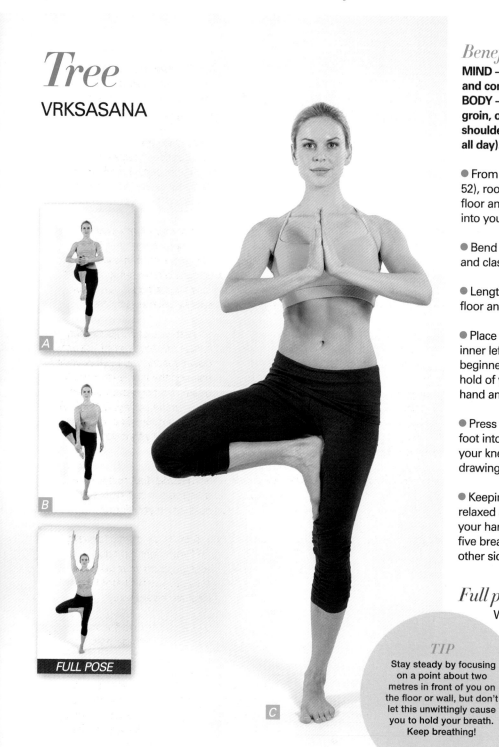

A

B

FULL POSE

C

Benefits

MIND – develops balance and concentration.
BODY – stretches your inner groin, opens your hips and shoulders (great if you sit all day).

● From Mountain pose (page 52), root your left foot into the floor and transfer your weight into your left leg.

● Bend right knee to your chest and clasp with both hands (A).

● Lengthen your tailbone to the floor and engage your belly.

● Place your right foot on your inner left thigh (or calf for beginners). If necessary, take hold of your foot with your right hand and place it (B).

● Press the sole of your right foot into your left thigh, turning your knee out to 90°, and drawing your tailbone down.

● Keeping your shoulders relaxed and chest lifted, bring your hands to prayer (C). Take five breaths and repeat on the other side.

Full pose

When you feel ready, move into the full pose by lifting your arms on an inhalation until parallel (or in a deep V) and holding for five breaths, shoulders relaxed.

TIP

Stay steady by focusing on a point about two metres in front of you on the floor or wall, but don't let this unwittingly cause you to hold your breath. Keep breathing!

Triangle
TRIKONASANA

Benefits

**MIND – mood-enhancing.
BODY – tones your waist,
and lengthens and tones
your legs.**

● From Mountain pose (page
52), step feet a leg's length
distance apart. Stretch your
arms out to the side, palms
down (A).

● Turn your left foot out 90°
and your right foot in 15°
degrees. On an inhalation,
torso and hips facing forward,
stretch your torso over your
left leg as far as you can.

● When you can't go further,
exhale and lower your left arm
down, resting the back of your
palm on the inside of your shin
or ankle, lifting your right arm
towards the ceiling. Either look
straight ahead (B) or down, or,
of it doesn't strain your neck,
look up (C).

● Root your feet to the floor,
lifting your inner arches to
strengthen your legs.

● Draw your left hip forward
and your right hip back,
and lengthen your tailbone
towards your left foot to
deepen the stretch.

● Take five to
10 breaths.

TIP
If your torso is
leaning forward,
practise against
a wall.

● Inhale, and
press down
through your
feet to come up.
Repeat on the
other side.

C

A

B

Reverse triangle
PARIVRITTI TRIKONASANA

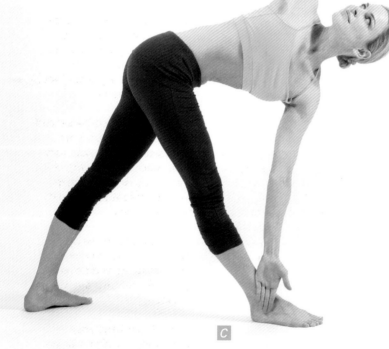

C

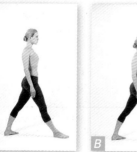

A   B

Benefits

**MIND – builds mental strength.
BODY – deeply tones your hamstrings, thighs and calves.**

● Step your feet a little less than a leg's length apart. Turn your right foot out 90° and your left foot in 45°.

● Square your hips to face the right and turn your torso to face the right (A). Inhale and lift your left arm over your head (B).

● Keeping your hips steady, feet rooting into the floor, exhale, and bend forwards from your hips to extend your torso out over your right leg.

● Place your left hand on your outside right shin or ankle, or on a block or the floor beside your right foot. Place your right hand on your lower back. Intermediate and advanced students: lift your right hand and twist your torso from your mid-body to look up at your hand (C).

● Lengthen your ribs away from your hips, lift your abdominals slightly.

● Keeping your hips level, draw your right hip slightly back and your left hip slightly forward to increase the stretch. Take five to 10 breaths.

TIP
Contract the muscles in your front thigh (quadriceps) to release the stretch in the backs of your thighs (hamstrings).

● Press down on your back foot to come up. Repeat on the other side.

Half-moon pose

ARDHA CHANDRASANA
(MODIFIED FOR BEGINNERS)

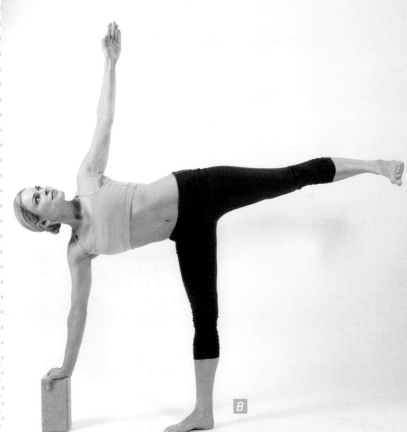

B

Benefits

MIND – fights tiredness and stress, centering and balancing.
BODY – aids digestion, tones your abs and outer thighs.

● Start in Triangle pose (page 57) on the right side. Place a block about a foot away from your right foot.

● On an inhalation, extend your left arm to the ceiling, bend your right leg and slide your left foot towards your right foot (A). If needed, rest your left arm on your hip. Raise your left leg behind you, parallel to the floor.

● Keeping your foot flexed and facing forward, place your right hand on the block. Turn your head to look up (B), or if this strains your neck, keep looking straight ahead. Hold for five breaths.

● Boost your balance by contracting your abs and supporting leg, and pointing your ankle towards the back of the room.

● To release, bend your supporting leg slightly before lowering your top leg to the floor.

● Repeat on the other side.

TIP
Most people balance better on one side than they do on the other. Try practising with your back a few inches from a wall until your balance improves.

Full pose
Intermediate and advanced: Perform the pose without the brick.

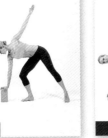

A

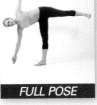

FULL POSE

Forward bend dynamic twist

PARIVRTTA UTTANASANA

Benefits

MIND – lifts mental fog.
BODY – tones your mid-spine and opens your shoulders.

- Start in Standing forward bend (page 54), feet hip-distance apart. Bend your knees deeply so your chest rests on your thighs and your hands are flat on the floor (A).

- Inhale, and stretch your right arm up to the ceiling, resting your left hand on the floor. At the same time, turn your torso and head to face the right (B).

- Feel the twist in your spine and the stretch in the right side of your body.

- Exhale, and release your right arm down, turning and relaxing your head and torso downward.

- Inhale, and extend your left arm up, repeating the process on the other side (C). Each move should be done with a single breath, so that you move with your breath.

- Repeat five times each side.

C

A   B

TIP

Keep both feet flat on the floor, knees and hips level so the twist comes from your waist. Don't be tempted to bring one knee forward to twist further.

High lunge

ASHVA SANCHALANASANA

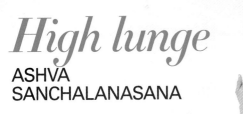

Benefits

**MIND – focusing and enlivening.
BODY – tones your inner and outer thighs and your tummy.**

● From Mountain pose (page 52), step your right leg back one leg's length, toes tucked under, ankle drawing backwards (A).

● Inhale, and stretch your arms over your head as you bend your left knee 90° and balance on the ball of your back foot.

● Sink your pelvis downwards, without it jutting forwards.

● Extend the heel of your back foot and put your weight into your back straight leg (B).

● Relax your shoulders, look straight ahead and take five breaths.

● On each inhalation, lengthen your torso and extend your tailbone down, and on each exhalation, sink deeper into your lunge. Take five to 10 breaths.

● Press down on your front foot to come up, and repeat on the other side.

Variation

Exhale, reach your arms to the sides and twist to the right, shoulders over your hips. Draw your back heel down and strengthen your legs. Contract your abs and root into your feet and look to your right. Take five breaths and repeat on the other side.

TIP
In standing postures, never bend your knee further than 90° – if you can't see your toes beneath your knee, you've gone too far!

B

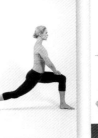

A

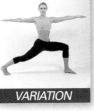

VARIATION

Crescent moon pose

ANJANEYASANA

Benefits

As for High lunge (page 61), plus opens your hips and chest and deeply stretches your thighs.

● Begin in Standing forward bend (page 54), knees bent (A).

● Step your right leg back, placing the top of your foot and your right knee on the floor. Beginners: keep your hands on your knees (B). Intermediate and advanced: lift your arms over your head so they are parallel.

● Open your chest, draw your hips and pelvis down and forward, and root your left foot into the floor.

● Draw in your abdominals. Keep your shoulders down and relaxed, and draw your shoulder blades together.

● Your lower back will want to take most of the arch, but open your back so your mid-spine takes most of your arch. Draw your tailbone down (C).

● Lengthen your neck but look forward. Take five deep breaths.

● To exit, exhale, bring your hands to the floor and step your right foot to your left, to standing forward bend. Repeat on the other side.

TIP

If you have sensitive knees, do this posture in a High lunge (page 61) instead of putting your knee on the floor, or place a folded blanket under the middle of your mat to cushion your knee.

Variation

Beginners: keep the toes of your straight leg tucked under.

C

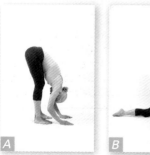

A

B

Warrior I
VIRABHADRASANA I

Benefits

MIND – strengthening and energising.
BODY – tones your legs, lower back and core muscles.

● Start in Mountain pose (page 52), feet hip-distance apart.

● Inhale, and step your right leg back a leg length's distance, back foot flat and turned 45° forward, front foot facing forward.

● Face your front foot, squaring your hips by drawing your left hip back and right hip forward (A).

● Inhale, raise your arms over your head, arms parallel, shoulders relaxed, and palms facing each other.

● Exhale, and bend your left knee to a 90° angle so it's over your ankle and sink your hips down (B).

● Root the outer edge of your back foot into the floor and lift the inner arches of both feet, feeling the stretch in your inner thigh. Look straight ahead.

● Take five to 10 deep breaths. Inhale, and straighten your left leg. Exhale, and press down into your right foot to come up. Repeat on the other side.

B

TIP
Intermediates: join your palms together. Advanced: lift your head and gaze up.

Variation
If you're having trouble keeping your the outer edge of your back foot rooted to the floor, rest the heel of your back foot on the edge of a block.

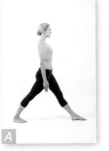

A

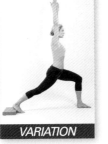

VARIATION

Warrior II

VIRABHADRASANA II

Benefits

MIND – builds mental strength.
BODY – tones your legs, arms and shoulders.

- Start in Mountain pose (page 52). Step your feet a little more than a leg's length distance apart.

- Turn your left foot out 90° and your right leg in 15°, so your left ankle points to the arch of your right foot.

- Keep your hips and torso facing forward.

- Inhale, and extend your arms out parallel to the floor, palms down. Extend your fingers and keep your shoulders soft.

- Lengthen your tailbone down and straighten your torso so your back doesn't over-arch (A).

- On an exhalation, bend your left knee to a right angle, shin perpendicular to the floor.

- Lift your inner arches, root down the outer edges of your feet and pull up the thigh muscle in your back leg for stability (B).

- Turn your head to gaze over your left arm. Hold for five to 10 deep breaths. Inhale, straighten your left leg and repeat on the other side.

B

TIP

Many people tend to lean forward in this posture. Your torso should rise directly upward from your hips, and your arms should feel like they are being stretched in opposite directions.

Variation

Lift your forward arm over your head and lean back over your straight leg. Root down into your feet. This is Reverse warrior.

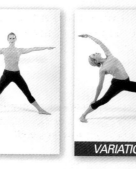

A   VARIATION

Warrior III
VIRABHADRASANA III

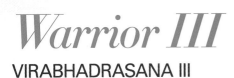

TIP
Contract your abdominals and keep the hip of your raised leg facing downwards for extra balance.

Benefits

MIND – focusing, builds balance.
BODY – tones your abs, hips and legs, and strengthens your ankles.

● Start in Mountain pose (page 52), feet hip-distance apart.

● Root the sole of your left foot down, lifting your inner arch. Inhale, transfer your weight to your left leg and lift your arms over your head.

● Exhale, lift your right leg and, leading with your chest and keeping your abdomen engaged, tilt your torso and arms forward (A).

● Rotate the outer edge of your right thigh down, so your hips are level.

● Keep the thigh muscles of your supporting leg strong, direct your right heel back, toes pointed down.

● Continue tilting forwards until your arms are straight out in front of you, palms facing each other and arms in a straight line with your head, torso and raised leg (B).

● Imagine your arms and raised leg stretching in opposite directions.

● Focus and take five to 10 breaths. Inhale to come up, then repeat on the other side.

Variation

Beginners: practise with your arms pressing against a wall or the sole of your back foot against a wall.

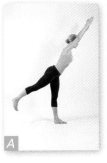

Extended side angle pose
PARSVAKONASANA

Benefits
MIND – grounding.
BODY – tones your outer thighs, improves your breathing and opens your chest, shoulders and hips.

● Start in Mountain pose (page 52) and step your feet a little more than a leg's length distance apart, left foot out 90° and right foot in 15°.

● On an in-breath, stretch your arms out to your sides, parallel to the floor, palms down.

● Exhale, and bend your left knee to a right angle, knee directly over your ankle.

● Inhale, and extend your torso over your left thigh without folding forward (A).

● Place your left hand on the floor, or on a block/brick, behind your left foot (B).

● Exhale and extend your right arm over your head, and look up at it (C).

● Press your left knee against your left arm.

● Root down into the outer edge of your back foot and engage your core.

● Take five to 10 deep breaths then repeat on the right leg.

TIP
Never let your knee turn inward when it's bent at right angles in this pose or in warrior I and warrior II.

Variation
Beginners: rest your front forearm on your thigh for extra support.

C

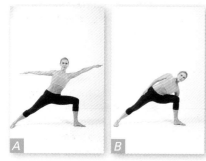

A

B

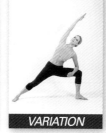

VARIATION

Revolved side stretch
PARSVOTTANASANA

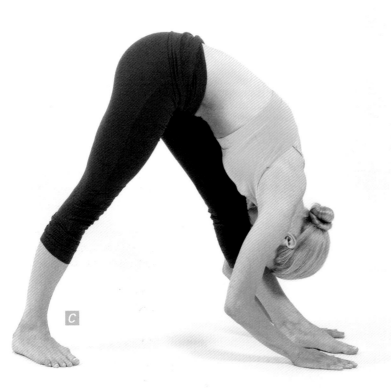

C

Benefits
MIND – calming.
BODY – tones and lengthens your hamstrings, strengthens your abdominals.

● From Mountain pose (page 52), step your feet three to four feet apart. Turn your left foot out 90° and your right foot in 45°.

● Turn your hips and torso to face the left, aligning your left heel with the right (A).

● Inhale, and lift your arms up over your head. Relax your shoulders down and draw your shoulder blades together.

● Firm your thighs, root your feet into the floor, and lift your inner arches.

● Exhale and, bending from your hips, extend your torso over your left leg, hands on your shin, ankle or the floor. Inhale, lengthen your spine and neck. Draw in your abdominals (B).

● Exhale, and curl your spine over your left leg, bending as far as is comfortable (C). Draw your left hip back and your right hip forward to deepen the hamstring stretch.

● Take five to 10 breaths then inhale, press into your feet to come up and repeat on the other side.

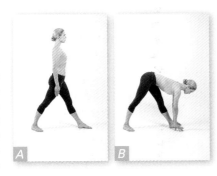

A   B

TIP
Try keeping one hand on your sacrum as you fold down to help keep your hips level.

Variation
For tight hamstrings, fold forward as far as comfortable and place your hands on your thighs or two blocks.

Wide-legged forward bend

PRASARITA PADOTTANASANA

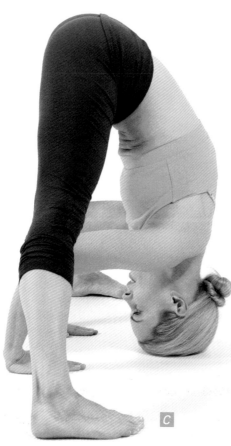

C

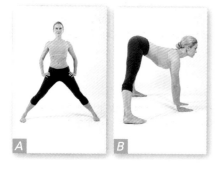

A

B

Benefits

Mind – calms a busy/tired brain. Body – tones your abdominals, strengthens and stretches your legs and spine, and conditions the small muscles in your feet.

● Step your feet about one-and-a-half leg length's distance apart, feet parallel. Hands on hips (A).

● Lift your inner arches and press the outer edges of your feet to the floor.

● Contract the muscles of your thighs without locking your knees.

● Inhale and, drawing your tailbone down, lengthen your spine and gently open your chest towards the ceiling. Look up without straining your neck.

● Exhale and, keeping your legs strong, hinge forward from your hips and bring your hands or finger tips to the floor. Inhale, lengthen your spine, look up (B).

● Exhale and, keeping your spine long, let your head relax down as far as is comfortable (C).

● Draw your tailbone up toward the ceiling and your inner groins away from each other. Take five to 10 deep breaths, keeping your neck relaxed.

● Inhale, straighten your arms and look forward.

● Exhale, bring your hands to your hip joints. Inhale, press your feet into the floor, contract your tummy and come up.

TIP

Contracting your quadriceps will help your hamstrings release, deepening the stretch.

Plank

KUMBHAKASANA

Benefits

MIND – builds focus.
BODY – great for warming your body. Tones your abs, bottom and upper body.

● Start on all fours, hands shoulder-width apart, directly under shoulders.

● Inhale, tuck your toes under and straighten your legs, so you're in a diagonal line from your head to your feet.

● Exhale, and tuck your chin in slightly, keep the back of your neck long.

● Engage your abdominal muscles, drawing them back towards your spine. Keep breathing evenly.

● Round your upper back and spread your shoulder blades apart.

● Root your palms into the floor, with your fingers fanning out, elbows straight but not locked. Take five to 10 breaths.

Variation

Beginners: keep your knees on the floor, tops of the feet facing down.

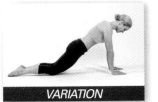

VARIATION

Side plank
VASISTHASANA
(INTERMEDIATE AND ADVANCED ONLY)

Benefits

As for Plank, but extra toning for your outer thighs and waistline.

● From Plank (page 69), inhale, press your left hand into the floor and roll over onto the outside edge of your left foot.

● Exhale, and stack your right ankle, hip and shoulder directly over your left ankle, hip and shoulder, balancing on your left hand and the outer edge of your left foot.

● Keep your left arm directly under your left shoulder, pressing into the floor.

● Keep the left side of your body lifted and strong, draw your abs to your spine and raise your hips.

● Inhale, and lift up your right arm, open your chest and look straight ahead. If this is too hard, try the variation below. Take five to 10 deep breaths, building up the length you hold the pose for. Repeat on the other side.

Variation

Beginners: bend your top leg and place your foot behind the knee of your straight leg. Keep hips lifted.

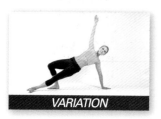

VARIATION

Squat
MALASANA

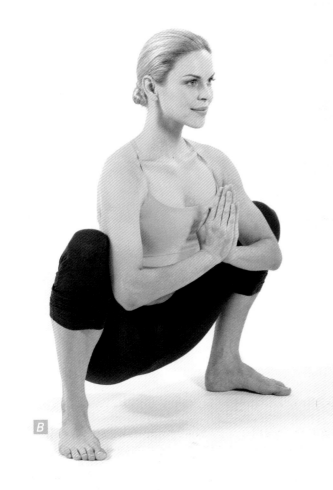

B

Benefits

MIND – builds focus and releases tension.
BODY – tones your abs and thighs, stretches your lower back and Achilles tendons.

- Start in Mountain pose (page 52), feet hip-distance apart, slightly turned out. Inhale, and place your hands in prayer (A).

- Exhale, and lower, bending your knees as if trying to sit down in a chair.

- Keeping your chest and shoulders open and your knees apart, lower your hips down further until your torso is between your knees.

- Separate your feet as much as you need to keep your ankles on the floor (you might need to turn them out a little more) and sink your heels into the floor.

- Press your elbows against your inner thighs and your hands together in prayer (B).

- Take five to 10 deep breaths, focusing your breath into your back.

- To come out, lower your body onto the floor.

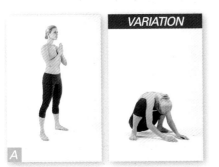

VARIATION

A

Variation

To relax deeply, place your hands on the floor in front of you, letting your head hang forward for 20 breaths.

TIP

If your feet come off the floor in this pose, place a block under each heel for extra support.

Downward-facing dog
ADHO MUKHA SVANASANA

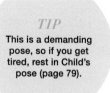

B

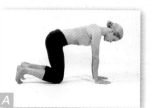

A

TIP

This is a demanding pose, so if you get tired, rest in Child's pose (page 79).

Benefits

MIND – relieves tiredness.
BODY – stretches your hamstrings, ankles and calves. Strengthens your arms, legs and shoulders.

● Kneel on all fours, legs hip-width apart, hands under your shoulders and fingers fanning out. Inhale.

● Exhale, and curl your toes under (A). Straighten your arms and extend your legs to raise your hips.

● Draw your shoulder blades back and relax your head.

● Draw in your abdominals, pull up your thigh muscles, press your thigh bones back and extend your heels toward the back of the room.

● Straighten your legs (beginners, keep legs bent) and point your tailbone to the ceiling.

● Extend your heels toward the floor – don't worry if they don't reach, focus on lifting your tailbone (B).

● Take five to 10 deep breaths, rooting your hands into the floor. Keep your thigh muscles strong and your head relaxed.

● To exit, bend your knees and come back to all fours.

Downward-facing dog splits
TRI PADA ADHO MUKHA SVANASANA

TIP
Keep your hands pressing into the floor and your hips level and facing down for maximum stretch.

Benefits
As Downward-facing dog (facing page), plus opens and tones your hips.

● From Downward-facing dog pose, inhale and bring your right leg straight up behind you, no higher than your hips, and flex your foot.

● Keep your hips squared to the floor and hold for two breaths, pressing your left foot into the floor. Exhale, release then repeat on the other side.

Variation
Make the pose dynamic by lowering your head and, on an exhalation, bending your knee so it almost reaches your head. Inhale as you reach your leg back up and lift your head back to the starting position. Repeat five to 10 times, then switch legs.

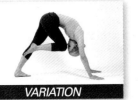

VARIATION

73

Shoulder stand

SALAMBA SARVANGASANA

Benefits
MIND – helps tiredness and stress.
BODY – stimulates your thyroid gland, and stretches your shoulders and back.

● Lie on your back. Exhale, firm your abdominals and lift your hips, so your legs are overhead, knees bent, and hips supported with your hands on your lower back (A).

● Tuck your shoulders under and bring your elbows closer together, hands on your back.

● Straighten your legs and bring them together – feel your legs working as though you're in Mountain pose.

● Bring your elbows closer together and point and extend your toes (B). Take up to 20 deep breaths.

● To exit, bend your knees, round your back and roll down slowly onto the floor, using your hands to support your back.

● Alternatively, lower into Plough pose (see facing page).

Variation
If your neck muscles are strained, hinge at your hips and fold your legs diagonally over your face – this is Half shoulder stand. If necessary, you can use a folded blanket under your shoulders for support.

B

TIP
If you're worried about having your feet in the air, practise with your feet against a wall until you feel more confident.

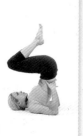

A

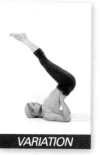

VARIATION

Plough
HALASANA

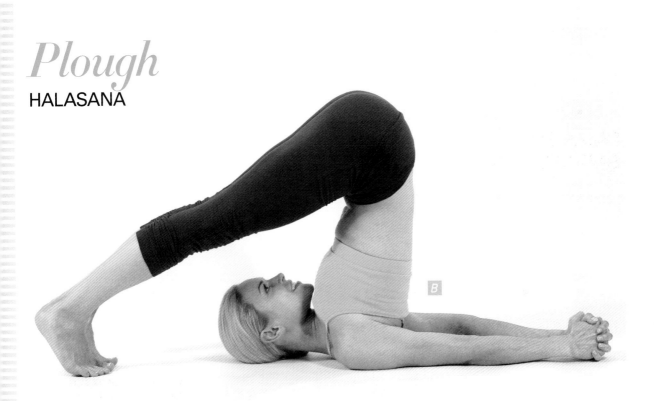

B

TIP
Push your heels
back in Plough,
to lengthen and
strengthen
your legs.

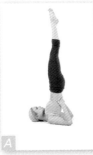

A

Benefits

As for Shoulder stand (facing page), plus stretches your spine and neck, and tones your tummy.

● From Shoulder stand (A), inhale deeply and, on the exhalation, lower your feet to the floor over your head, toes tucked under. Still supporting your back with your hands.

● Rest your toes on the floor. Keep your torso lifted and your shoulder blades drawn together underneath you.

● Stretch your arms out behind you and interlace your fingers (B). Take 10-20 steady breaths,

keeping your torso straight (don't let it collapse).

● To come down, support your back with your hands, lift your feet off the floor and slowly roll down one vertebra at a time until you are lying flat.

Variation

If lowering your feet to the floor is difficult, rest your feet on a chair or against a wall. Support your back with your hands.

Supported headstand

SALAMBA SIRSASANA

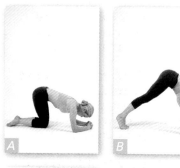
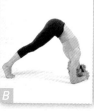

A

B

C

D

TIP

Contracting your core muscles and focusing on your breath will help your balance. And if you fold your mat twice, you can create a cushion effect for your head.

Variation

Beginners: practise against a wall to help you sense what it feels like to stack your hips over your shoulders. Over time, move further away from the wall.

Benefits

MIND – calms and increases concentration.
BODY – improves circulation, energy, and shoulder, arm and core strength.

- On your hands and knees, bring your forearms to the floor, elbows under your shoulders, and fingers clasped with thumbs touching and resting on your index fingers (A).

- Bend forward and place the crown of your head onto the floor against your hands. Keep your neck long and shoulders down.

- Straighten your legs, pointing your hips up and balancing on your toes (B).

- Slowly walk your feet forward, contracting your abdominals. Feel your hips stacking over your shoulders. Your forearms should be taking most of your weight.

- Breathe steadily. When your hips are over your shoulders, contract your abs, bend your knees and lift your knees toward your chest and raise your hips (C).

- When your hips and torso are in a line, straighten your legs (D).

- Stay for 10-20 breaths to 10 minutes.

- To come down, exhale and slowly bring your legs to the floor. Rest in Child's pose (page 79).

Legs up the wall
VIPARITA KARANI

Benefits

MIND – deeply relaxing, rejuvenates a tired mind.
BODY – relaxes your lower back, relieves tired legs.

● Place a bolster or folded blanket on the floor one to two inches away from a wall.

● Lie on the edge of the bolster or blanket in a foetal position, the bottom of your buttocks against the wall (A).

● Slowly roll onto your back so you're lying in the middle of the bolster, your lower back resting on it with your legs and hips against the wall.

● Exhale and rest the backs of your legs against the wall, arms out to your sides, palms facing up (B).

● Stay here for 20 breaths or up to 15 minutes. With every exhalation, feel your body sink deeper into the floor.

● To release, bend your knees, turn over and rest on your blanket or bolster for a moment before sitting up.

Variation

If you have tight hamstrings, move the folded blanket or bolster further from the wall for a gentler lift in the legs.

TIP
If you find your legs fanning apart, tie them together at the thighs with a belt or scarf.

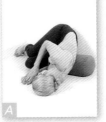

Hero pose
VIRASANA

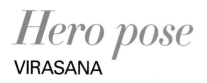

Benefits

MIND – centering.
BODY – helps digestion, and stretches your thighs.

● Sit on your heels, release the tops of your thighs and lift your spine.

● Keeping your knees together, pull your waist back and up, and lengthen the back of your neck, pointing the crown of your head to the ceiling.

● Bring your hands together in prayer, and roll your shoulders back and down to expand your chest. Focus inward and take five to 20 steady breaths.

● To release, place your hands on the floor beside your legs, lean onto one hip and extend your opposite leg, then lean to the other side and extend your other leg, so you're sitting in staff pose (page 82).

Modification

Beginners: place a block or rolled blanket between your heels and bottom. If your ankles hurt, roll up a soft blanket and place it under them before you start.

Variation

Extended hero pose – interlace your fingers and extend your arms over your head for a delicious arm and shoulder stretch.

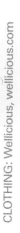

CLOTHING: Wellicious, wellicious.com

VARIATION

Child's pose
BALASANA

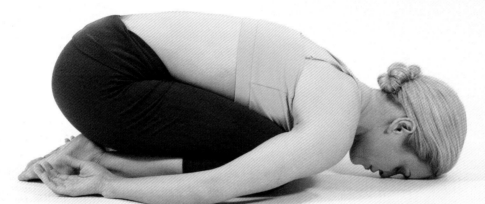

TIP
If your belly or bust is in the way, or if you want a deeper hip opener, take your knees further apart but keep your big toes touching.

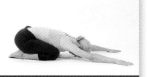
VARIATION

Benefits

MIND – stress-relieving, soothing, calming.
BODY – great for bloating or gas. Stretches and soothes your lower back and upper body, and opens your hips.

- Kneel down with your bottom resting on your heels and the tops of your feet on the floor. Inhale.

- Exhale, and move your torso forward so it folds over your thighs and your forehead rests on the floor. If it doesn't reach the ground, rest your forehead on a book or block.

- Rest your arms by the sides of your legs, or cross them on the floor in front of you and make a pillow to rest your forehead on.

- Relax your head and neck, and feel your shoulders sink down to the floor.

- Breathe slowly and deeply for one to five minutes, directing your breath into your back ribs. Relax your entire torso on each exhalation.

Variation

For a more active pose, stretch your arms in front of you, fingertips pressing into the floor.

Cobbler poses

BADDHA KONASANA

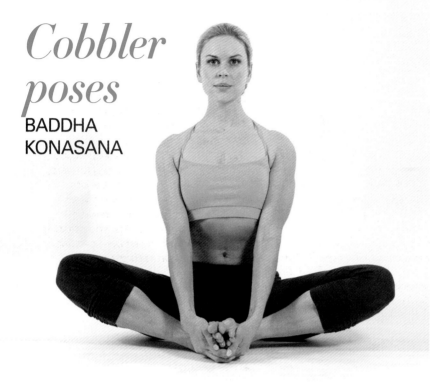

Benefits

MIND – eases anxiety, mild depression and tiredness.
BODY – stretches your inner thighs, knees and groin. Stimulates your circulation, stretches your spine and tones your abdominals.

Version 1:
Sitting upright (classic pose)

● Start seated. Inhale, bend your knees and draw your feet towards your groin, with your soles together, as close to your pelvis as is comfortable. Exhale.

● Inhale, and hold your feet, ankles or shins. Lengthen the crown of your head upwards. Take five to 10 breaths or hold for up to five minutes.

Version 2:
Folding forward with straight back (enlivening)

● From version one, inhale and lengthen your spine.

● Exhale, and slowly tilt forward from your pelvis with your spine straight (as though you're trying to bring your navel to your feet).

● Inhale, lengthen your spine, then exhale and tilt forward from your hips as far as is comfortable, keeping your shoulders down. Take five to 10 breaths and release.

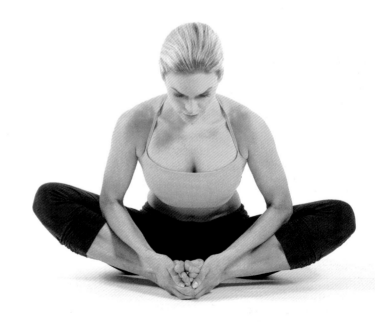

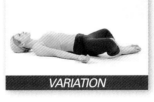

Version 3: Coming forward with rounded back (calming)

● From version one, gently clasp your hands around the back of your head and bring your chin to your chest.

● Round your spine, bringing your head and hands forward, pointing your mid-back to the ceiling and letting your head hang to wherever is comfortable. Rest your clasped hands behind your head and take five to 10 deep breaths.

Version 4: Lying supine (relaxing)

● From version one, exhale, round your pelvis inward so your tailbone extends down, firm your abs and lay back, supporting yourself with your elbows until your body is supine.

● Stretch your arms out to 45° and breathe. Ensure your hips are only open as far as is comfortable.

Variation

If your hips are tight or your knees high off the ground, move your feet further away from your body. If you have sore knees, place cushions or blocks beneath them.

VARIATION

TIP

To make version four even more relaxing, place a bolster or two folded blankets at the base of your back, and rest your back, shoulders and head on them. Stay in the pose for up to five minutes, breathing deeply into the side of your ribcage.

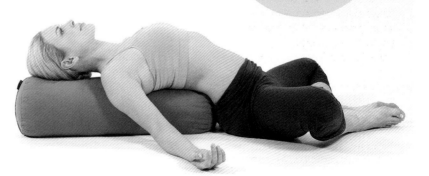

Staff pose
DANDASANA

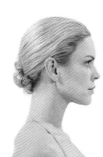

Benefits

MIND – focusing.
BODY – improves posture, stretches your back, opens your shoulders and chest, and tones your arms and upper thighs.

- Sit on the floor with your torso straight, legs together and extended in front of you, toes pointing upward.

- Sit toward the front of your sitting bones – try pulling the fleshy bits of your bottom out to the sides, so you feel your sitting bones on the floor.

- Press the backs of your thighs and your sitting bones into the floor, and rotate your thighs slightly inward toward each other, so your legs remain active, knees facing upward.

- Root your hands down beside (or a little behind) your hips, keeping your shoulders down and relaxed. Look straight ahead, drawing in your chin slightly to make your neck long.

- Flex your feet and extend your heels forward.

- Inhale, and lengthen your torso. Imagine being stretched from your pubic bone upwards through the crown of your head. Exhale.

- Take five to 10 deep breaths.

Variation

If you find yourself leaning back in this posture or find it difficult to perform, sit with a blanket or block under your buttocks or sit against a wall to keep your back straight.

Sitting forward bend
PASCHIMOTTANASANA

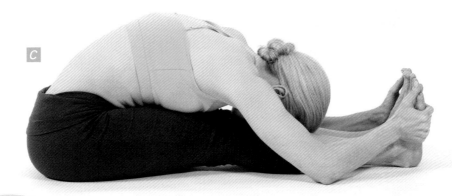

C

TIP
Sitting on a block or cushion helps release the stretch. If you are extra stiff, use a rolled up blanket under your knees and keep them slightly bent.

Benefits
MIND – helps stress, headache and tiredness.
BODY – stretches your spine, shoulders and hamstrings.

● Follow the directions for Staff pose (see facing page). Inhale, and raise your arms over your head, contract your abdominals (A).

● Exhale, and fold your torso forwards from your hips, extending your spine as far as you can. Keep your head and spine aligned.

● With your chest open and shoulders relaxed, gently take hold of your toes, sides of feet or shins with your hands. Look forward to your toes, not down (B).

● If you're holding your toes or feet, bend your elbows to the side (C).

● Take five to 10 breaths. With each inhalation, lift and lengthen your torso and with each exhalation, release further into the stretch.

Variation
If you're a beginner or are straining to reach your feet with a straight back, hold a belt around your feet to come forward.

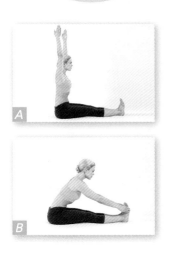

A

B

One leg bent sitting extension

JANU SIRASANA

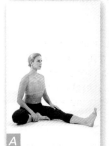

TIP
For really tight hamstrings, keep your extended leg a little bent (you'll still feel a stretch).

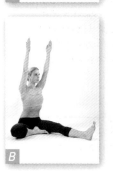

Benefits

MIND – helps tiredness and headache, lifts mood.
BODY – stretches your spine, inner thighs and hamstrings.

● Sit with your legs in front of you. Inhale, and bend your right leg, placing the sole of your foot to the inside of your left thigh. Exhale (A).

● Inhale, lift your arms and turn your torso to face forward. You should feel a slight twist in your mid-spine. Keep your hips level and facing forward (B).

● Exhale, and extend forward from your hips, taking hold of your foot, shin or thigh (C).

● If you have tight hamstrings or hips, use a belt around the ball of your foot and draw closer to your leg (don't pull yourself forward).

● Look at your big toes, maintaining length in your spine and keeping shoulders relaxed and down. Keep your neck extended. On each inhalation extend your spine, and on each exhalation stretch forward.

● Take five to 10 deep breaths. Feel a stretch in your left hamstring and the right side of your body. Repeat on the other side.

Variation

If your bent knee is high off the floor, sit on a block or cushion. For sore knees, use a cushion or block beneath your bent knee for support.

Seated wide-legged forward bend
UPAVISTHA KONASANA

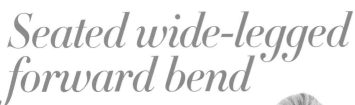

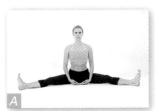

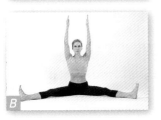

TIP
Make sure you don't get caught up in having your legs too far apart in this posture. Only separate them as far as is comfortable to maintain alignment.

Benefits
MIND – deeply relaxing.
BODY – stretches your inner thighs and lower back, opens your chest and tones your legs.

- Sit with your legs apart in a V-shape. Pull out the flesh from under your bottom, so your sitting bones make contact with the floor and your spine is upright (A).

- Inhale, and draw your arms over your head, keeping your shoulders down. Root your pelvis down and lengthen your spine upwards (B).

- Exhale, and tilt forward from your hips, keeping your spine straight, knees facing up.

- Place your hands flat on the floor in front of you, shoulder-width apart. Keep your neck long and your chin slightly tucked in.

- Keep your knees and toes pointing upwards, heels extending forward, feet flexed and thigh muscles engaged and rooted to the floor (C). Don't rotate your legs inward or outward to come forward further.

- Take five to 10 breaths. Keep your tailbone long and rooted to the floor to help release the inner thigh stretch. Don't sacrifice alignment to come forward with your hands.

Variation
If your back is rounded, sit on a blanket or block, to help tilt your pelvis forward onto your sitting bones.

Seated wide-legged side stretch

PARIVRTTA UPAVISTHA KONASANA

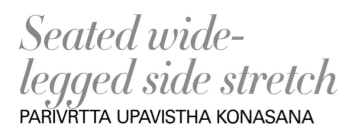

C

TIP
There is a tendency to slouch the shoulders and torso forward. Keep your chest open and facing forward as you stretch sideways, your top arm in line with your ear, and your ear facing up.

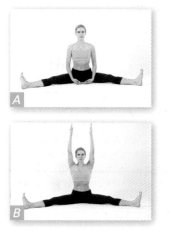

A

B

Benefits

As with previous pose, plus a deep waist and diaphragmatic stretch which improves breathing.

● Sit with your legs wide apart in a V-shape. Pull out the flesh from under your bottom, so your sitting bones make contact with the floor and your spine is upright (A).

● Inhale, draw your arms over your head, root your pelvis down and lengthen your spine upwards (B).

● Exhale, and stretch your torso sideways, taking your left big toe with your left hand or resting your hand or forearm inside your left knee or shin, arm bent.

● Inhale and extend your right arm over your right ear, keeping your neck long and relaxed and your shoulders open. Rotate your right shoulder back and your left shoulder forward, so shoulders remain open (C). Exhale.

● Keep the backs of your legs grounded to the floor, and your feet flexing upwards.

● Take five deep breaths, feeling a deep stretch in the side of your body. Repeat on the other side.

Easy cross-legged pose
SUKHASANA

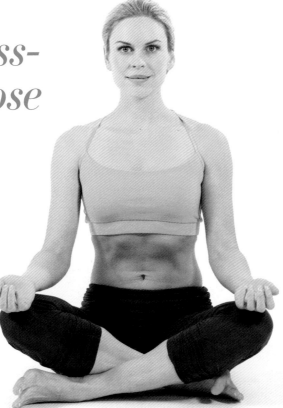

TIP
If you're sitting for longer than five breaths in this pose, alternate the cross of your legs to get an even stretch.

Benefits

MIND – calming, stress-relieving.
BODY – strengthens your back. Stretches your knees and ankles.

● Sitting on the floor, cross your legs in front of you (if your back is rounding or straining, or your knees are above your hips, use a block, cushion or blanket).

● Slip each foot under the opposite knee, so there is a gap between your feet and your pelvis.

● Lengthen your tailbone towards the floor and extend your spine and the crown of your head upwards.

● Rest the backs of your hands on your knees or one on top of the other in your lap, facing upwards.

● Sit in this pose for five to 10 breaths or longer in meditation (see page 35).

Variation

For a wonderful outer thigh stretch, inhale your arms up and, as you exhale, tilt your torso forward from the hips, bringing your hands to the floor in front of you, shoulder-width apart. Take five breaths. Extend your spine and press your buttocks into the floor on each inhalation, and on each exhalation, release further into the stretch. Come up, change the cross of your legs and repeat.

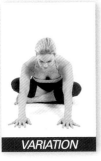

VARIATION

Boat pose
NAVASANA

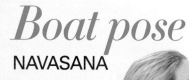

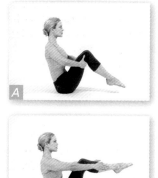

TIP
To balance on your tailbone, use your abdominals for support, keep your chest lifted and open, shoulders back and relaxed, lower back lifted.

Benefits

MIND – focusing and stress-relieving.
BODY – deeply tones your tummy muscles and spine, and aids digestion.

● Sit on the floor, with your legs out straight in front of you.

● On an inhalation, bend your knees and lift your feet off the floor a few inches. Place your hands on the backs of your thighs. Engage your abdominals and lean back so you balance on your tailbone. This is stage one of the posture (A). Absolute beginners can practise this by taking five breaths here.

● Now, lift your feet and keep your knees bent so your shins are parallel to the floor. Continue to balance on your tailbone. If you are comfortable in this position, straighten your arms and hold them

parallel to the floor – this is stage two. Intermediate students can practise this by taking five breaths here (B).

● Advanced students: holding the backs of your thighs, straighten your legs in front of you, so your torso and legs are at a 45° angle from the floor, toes gently pointing, feet relaxed, abdominals fully engaged.

● If you feel strong and supple, take your arms away from your thighs and stretch them out parallel to the floor, palms facing each other (C). Take five breaths and release. Repeat up to five times.

Cobra
BHUJANGASANA

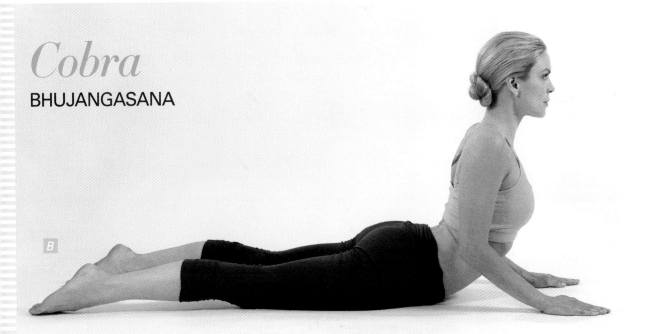

B

TIP
As you come up, imagine someone pulling you forward, then upward, from the crown of your head.

Benefits

MIND – refreshing, invigorating.
BODY – firms your bottom, shoulders and chest, stretches spine and core.

● Lie on your stomach, legs straight, with your feet together, facing down.

● Place your palms on the floor below your shoulders.

● Hug your elbows towards your body to open your chest.

● Press the tops of your feet, thighs and pubic bone into the floor (A).

● Inhale, and stretch the crown of your head and chest forward, then up, keeping your neck long. Raise your head and shoulders, and lift your torso as far as is comfortable and arch your back.

● Open your chest, pointing your sternum up and firming your tummy

muscles toward your spine, shoulder blades drawing together.

● Continue pressing your pubic bone, feet and thighs into the floor.

● Look forward by raising your eyes. Don't flop your neck backwards (this is dangerous). Keep your neck long, with the crown of your head pointing upwards (B). Take five to 10 breaths.

Variation

Try using no hands as you come up, to help strengthen your lower back. Just let your hands hover above the floor while you gently arch upwards. You might only come up a few inches – that's fine. This pose isn't about how high you can come – less is more!

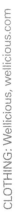

A

Locust
SALABHASANA

TIP
Imagine the crown of your head and your feet extending away from each other, then upward, so you are stretching your entire body before lifting your torso and legs.

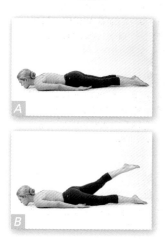

Benefits

MIND – stress-relieving, energising.
BODY – works your hamstrings and buttocks, stretches your spine and core. Improves your posture.

● Lie prone, your chin resting on the mat, feet facing down, arms at your sides, palms facing up. Take a few centering breaths (A).

● Inhale and lift one leg up, firm it, turn it inwards, stretch it back (B) and exhale to lower it. Repeat with your other leg.

● Keeping your legs firm, draw your tailbone toward your heels and press your pubic bone into the mat.

● Inhale and, keeping your neck long, lift both thighs, head and chest away from the floor.

● Stretch your hands towards your feet (C).

● Take five breaths and release on an exhalation. Make a pillow with one hand over the other and rest your head on your hands, face to one side. Repeat three to five times.

Variation

Beginners: build up lower back and glute strength by keeping your chin on the floor and your hands under your pubic bone for support. Raise one leg at a time and hold for 30 seconds each, then lift both legs together and hold.

Bow

DHANURASANA
(INTERMEDIATE AND ADVANCED ONLY)

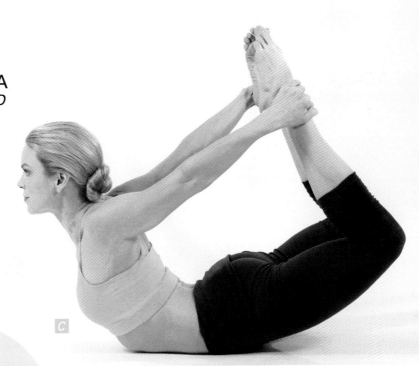

TIP

With each inhalation, lengthen the crown of your head upwards and extend your lower back. With each exhalation, open your chest a little further and draw your thighs, knees and feet up and towards each other.

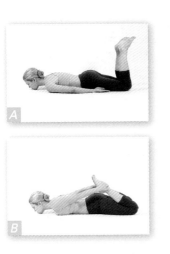

Benefits

MIND – energising, mood-lifting.
BODY – firms and lengthens your arms, chest, core, hips, legs, back and bottom.

● Lie flat on your tummy, chin resting on the floor

● Bend your knees so your shins are perpendicular to the floor (A).

● Inhale, and extend your right arm back toward your feet. Exhale, and release. Repeat with your left hand.

● Inhale, and extend both arms back toward your feet, taking hold of your ankles or shins (B). Exhale.

● Inhale, press your pubic bone into the mat, the fronts of your feet into your hands and lift your heels away from your bottom, toward the ceiling. Raise your thighs. This should automatically open your chest and lift your head and chest off the floor.

● Press your tailbone and pubic bone into the mat. Draw your shoulders down, and open and lift your chest, pointing your sternum upwards (C).

● Keeping your breath steady, focus on bringing your knees, ankles and feet closer together, so you feel an opening in your entire body. Take five to 10 breaths.

Variation

If this pose hurts your pubic bone, put a thinly folded blanket under it before you begin.

Camel

USTRASANA

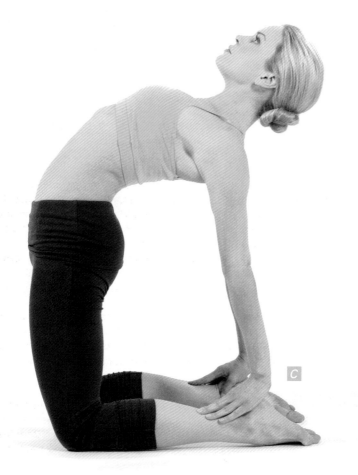

C

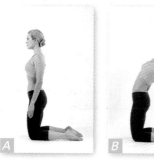

A

B

Benefits

MIND – energising.
BODY – deeply opens your abdominals, chest and shoulders, firms and lengthens your thighs and hip flexors.

● Kneel upright on a mat, thighs hip-width apart, tops of your feet against the mat (A).

● Inhale, lift your chest and torso, stretch your left arm over your head and rest it on your left ankle, fingers pointing to your knees (B). Exhale.

● Inhale, and repeat with your right hand. Keep your neck straight, without straining.

● Exhale, and open your chest and shoulders, lifting your sternum gently upwards.

● Keep your neck long, chin tucked in slightly. Advanced practitioners: take your head back and look up if this doesn't strain your neck (C).

● Draw your tailbone under and pubic bone upward to release the stretch in your thighs and abdomen.

● Take five to 10 deep breaths, opening your chest and hips. To release, exhale into kneeling, then Child's pose (page 79).

TIP

There is a tendency to collapse your legs back in this pose. If you do this, practise with the tops of your thighs against a wall and, as you move into the pose, press your thighs gently against the wall.

Variation

Beginners: tuck your toes under or place an brick either side of your feet to rest your hands on.

Bridge

SETUBHANDA
SARVANGASANA

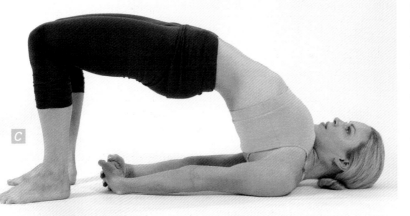

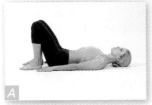

A

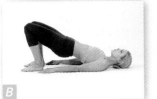

B

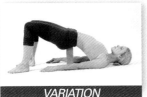

VARIATION

C

Benefits

MIND – lifts tiredness and mood, relieves stress, helps insomnia. BODY – stretches your core and back, firms back and inner thighs.

● Lie on your back, knees bent with feet hip-width apart, thighs parallel and shins vertical (A).

● Inhale, and roll your pelvis inwards and upwards, slowly lifting your bottom and spine off the floor, one vertebra at a time until your weight is resting on your shoulders (B). Exhale.

● Inhale, and reach your hands under your body and clasp them. Breathe steadily, ensuring your thighs remain parallel, knees directly over your ankles – don't let them splay outwards. Beginners take five to 10 breaths here.

● Intermediate and advanced practitioners: tuck your shoulders under and squeeze your shoulder blades together to further open your chest.

● On an inhalation, press firmly into the soles of your feet and elevate your pelvis further (C). Take five to 10 deep breaths.

● To release, exhale and slowly roll down, one vertebra at a time, beginning from your upper spine.

TIP

To keep your thighs parallel and working, place a brick or thick book between your knees.

Variation

For a restorative version, place a brick on the floor under your lower back and rest.

Pigeon pose
EKA PADA RAJAKAPOTASANA

B

Benefits

MIND – energising.
BODY – opens your hips, stretches your outer thighs, lengthens your spine.

- Start on all fours, knees beneath hips, hands beneath shoulders (A).

- Lift your right knee and place it a few inches behind your right wrist.

- Gently slide back the left leg, straightening it out.

- Place your right heel in front of your left hip (as you progress, or experienced students, move the heel of your bent leg further from the front of your hip to help open your hips).

- Inhale, and lengthen your torso by extending the crown of your head to the ceiling, pressing your fingers into the floor and chin to your chest (B).

- On an exhalation, lean your torso over your bent leg and relax down into folded pigeon pose (use a bolster if you don't reach the floor). Take a few deep breaths (C).

- Ensure your weight is even on both hips, don't tilt to one side.

- On an inhalation, press your palms into the floor and lift your torso, drawing your tailbone down and core upward and pressing your hips into the mat. Exhale.

- Inhale, root your palms to the floor and lift your chest, drawing back the shoulder blades and straightening your arms as much as is comfortable. Look ahead and take five to 10 deep breaths.

- Release the pose by pressing your hands into the floor, lifting your hips and moving back to hands and knees. Repeat on the other side.

Modification

If the hip of your bent leg is lifting off the floor, place a block under it.

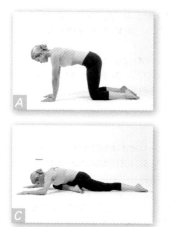

A

C

Wheel

URDHVA DHANURASANA
*(INTERMEDIATE AND
ADVANCED ONLY)*

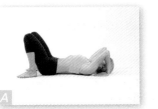

B

A

TIP
Straighten your
legs and arms as
much as you can
in the pose and
imagine being lifted
up by the navel.

Benefits

MIND – soothes stress, increases energy.
**BODY – strengthens your whole body, especially your thighs, shoulders,
arms, wrists and spine.**

● Lie on your back, knees bent and
heels as close as is comfortable to
your buttocks.

● Place your palms on the floor
beside your shoulders, fingers
towards your feet, elbows close to
your body, pointing upwards (A).

● Inhale, press your hands and feet
firmly into the floor and lift your hips
up and back. Lift your head and
place the crown of your head on
the floor. Your forearms should
be parallel to the floor, elbows
shoulder-width apart. Exhale.

● Inhale, and straighten your arms

and legs as much as is comfortable,
lifting your body (B).

● Look back and relax your neck,
taking five to eight deep breaths.

● Lower gently by bending your
knees and arms, and repeat up to
five times (advanced only).

Variation

Get an even better stretch by lifting
your heels off the floor once you are
in the full pose. Extend your chest,
stretch up through your lower back
and feel your abs tightening. Lower
your heels as you exhale.

Easy cross-legged twist
PARIVRITTA SUKHASANA

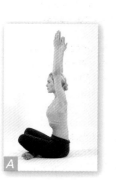

B

CLOTHING: Wellicious, wellicious.com

TIP
As you hold the twist, lengthen your spine on each inhalation and move further into your twist on each exhalation. The longer your spine is on the in-breath, the more flexible it will be on the out-breath.

Benefits

MIND – better focus.
BODY – stretches your mid-spine, tones your abdomen and waist.

● Begin in Easy cross-legged pose, each foot under the opposite knee. If you're leaning back in the pose or your knees are sitting high above your hips, sit on a block or cushion.

● Inhale, lengthen your spine and raise your arms up over your head until they are parallel (A).

● Exhale, turn your chest to the left, placing the back of your right palm on the outside of your left knee and your left palm behind your buttocks, flat or on your fingertips.

● Use your right hand to gently lever the twist but don't pull, most of the twist should come from your mid-back (B).

● Keep your shoulders down, your chin drawn in slightly and look over your left shoulder without straining your neck. Your hips should remain square and facing forward.

● Take 10 deep breaths. Release and repeat on the other side.

Mermaid pose
BHARADVAJASANA

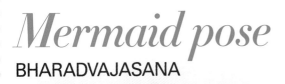

TIP
Lift and twist from your lower and mid-spine. Don't let your hips and pelvis come forward, keep them level and in contact with the floor.

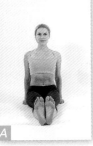

A

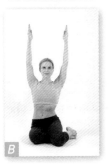

B

Benefits

MIND – centering.
BODY – stretches your lower spine, neck and shoulders.

● Sit in Staff pose (A). Bend your knees, shift your body weight to your right hip and bring both feet to your left buttock, top left foot resting on the arch of your right.

● Inhale, lift both arms up (B) and, on an exhale, twist from your mid-spine to turn your chest toward your right hip.

● Reach your left palm to the outside of your right knee, your right hand behind you on your fingertips (C). Hold for five to 10 breaths.

● With each inhalation, lengthen your spine upwards as though

someone is lifting you from the crown of the your head. With each exhalation, move your chest further to the right and your right shoulder toward the back of your body.

● Keep your chin tucked in and look behind you without straining.

● To release, turn your head forward first, follow with your chest, then your hips. Repeat on the other side.

Variation
If one side of your buttocks is coming off the floor, put a cushion or blanket under it until it's level.

Seated spine twist
MARICHYASANA C

B

TIP
Keep your straight leg engaged (there will be a tendency for it to splay outwards). Both hips should remain on the floor, level and facing forwards.

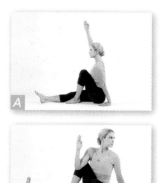

A

VARIATION

Benefits
MIND – stimulating.
BODY – tones your abs and waist, and strengthens your spine.

● Begin in Staff pose (page 82). Bend your left knee, foot rooted flat to the floor. If possible, take your foot as close as possible to your buttock, about two to three inches from your upper left thigh.

● Inhale and lift your right arm up (A). Exhale and turn your chest toward the left, wrapping your right arm around your left knee and placing your left hand behind you, fingertips or palm on the floor (B).

● Take 10 breaths, lengthening your spine on each inhalation and twisting a little further on each exhalation. Keep your chest expanded, shoulders back and down.

● Look to the left, without straining your neck.

● Release by first turning your head to look forward, releasing your arms and then turning to the front. Repeat on the other side.

Variation
Intermediate or advanced: take your right elbow to the outside of your left knee and open the twist further by pushing your elbow against your left thigh and looking back.

Reclining twist
SUPTA MATSYENDRASANA

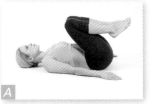

A

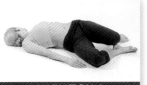

VARIATION A

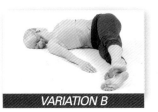

VARIATION B

Benefits

MIND – relaxing, soothing, stress-relieving.
BODY – deeply stretches your waist, soothes your spine and lower back.

● Lie on your back, knees bent to your chest (A).

● Take both bent legs over to the right, stacking your knees and feet over each other. If needed, you can use your right hand on your left knee to encourage it to the floor.

● Straighten your arms and take them out to the sides, no higher than shoulder height (B).

● Look to the left. Feel the stretch through your hips and waist as you take 10 deep breaths. Release and switch sides.

Variation A

For a stretch to the lower waist, begin with knees bent and feet on the floor, hip-width apart under your knees. Drop your knees to the right, head to the left, relaxing your feet onto their sides. Repeat on the other side, with feet in the same place.

Variation B

Advanced and intermediate: for a deeper stretch, once in the main pose, lengthen your legs, stacking one straight leg over the other, and look to your left.

Happy baby
ANANDA BALASANA

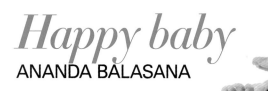

B

Benefits

MIND – uplifting and stress-relieving.
BODY – stretches your inner and outer thighs, and lower back.

● Begin lying on your back. Bend both knees deeply, slightly wider than your body, feet flexed and facing the ceiling (A).

● Take your outer feet with your hands.

● Bend your knees toward your armpits. Feel the stretch and deep release in your lower back.

● Draw in your chin to lengthen your neck, keep your shoulders down and relaxed, and point your tailbone forward to lengthen your spine (B).

● Take 10-20 breaths, rocking side to side if it feels comfortable. Release your feet to the floor.

Variation

If you can't easily hold your feet with your hands, hold the backs of your shins. Alternatively, wrap a scarf or strap around the ball of each foot and hold onto that wherever is comfortable. Over time, you can move further up the strap until you're holding your feet.

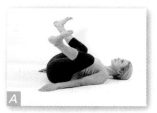

A

Reclining head-to-toe sequence
SUPTA PADANGUSTHASANA

B

TIP

If it's a strain to take your toe in your fingers, take your shin instead, or use a strap wrapped around the ball of your foot.

Benefits

MIND – calming, relaxing.
BODY – deeply stretches your hamstrings, groin and inner thighs.

● Lie flat. Bend your left knee and hug it to your chest with your arms. Take a couple of breaths here.

● Inhale and straighten your left leg, taking your big toe with your fingers (hold your shin if you can't reach).

● Keep your shoulders down and relaxed. Ensure your straight right leg remains engaged and rotating inwards, knee facing up, toes pointing up and heel flexing forward (A).

● Beginners: if this feels strained and causes your lower back to lift off the floor, bend your right knee and place your foot flat on the floor.

● Now, externally rotate your left leg so your toes point out to the side. Slowly lower your leg to the

left side as far as is comfortable, without your left leg and thigh tipping over (B).

● Turn your head to the right, relaxing your shoulders and neck, lower leg remaining engaged.

● Keep your right hip down (it will want to rise). You can gently guide your right hip down with your right hand or release your arm straight out to the right. Take five breaths.

● Bring your leg back to the centre and gently release. Repeat on the other side.

Variation

Beginners: bend your right leg, and using a strap around your left foot, extend it gently towards your chest.

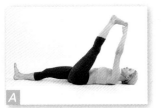

A

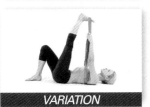

VARIATION

Knees to chest

APASANA

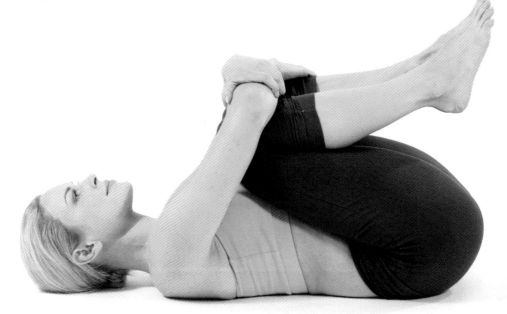

TIP
If you have tight knees, try holding the backs of your thighs instead of your knees.

Benefits

MIND – deeply relaxing, promotes sleep.
BODY – stretches out the spine.

● Lie flat. If you have a tight or sensitive neck, rest your head on a block or folded blanket.

● Exhale and, keeping your legs together, bend your knees to your chest.

● Hold your shins with your hands, just below your knees, and draw them into your chest. Hug your knees with your arms if comfortable.

● On each inhalation, open your back and allow your legs to move slightly away.

● On each exhalation, hug your knees closer to your chest.

● Take 10-20 deep breaths.

Variation

If it's comfortable, gently rock slightly from side to side while in this pose for a delicious massage to your lower back.

Corpse
SAVASANA

Benefits

MIND – invigorating, deeply relaxing.
BODY – stabilises breathing, and helps your muscles relax and absorb the benefits of your practice.

● From Staff pose (page 82), use your hands to push the flesh of your bottom out to the sides.

● Bend your knees, feet hip-distance apart, and hold the tops of your shins with your hands.

● Lower your torso back, placing your forearms and palms on the floor and leaning back on your elbows.

● Lower your torso to the floor one vertebra at a time until the back of your head rests on the floor.

● Turn your palms to face the ceiling, arms about a foot away from your torso. Straighten your legs and let your feet relax out to the sides.

● Close your eyes, relax your whole body and allow your breath to slow as you totally let go. Stay in this pose up to 10 minutes.

Modifications

If you have a tight lower back, place two rolled blankets under your knees. If your neck feels uncomfortable, place a block under your head.

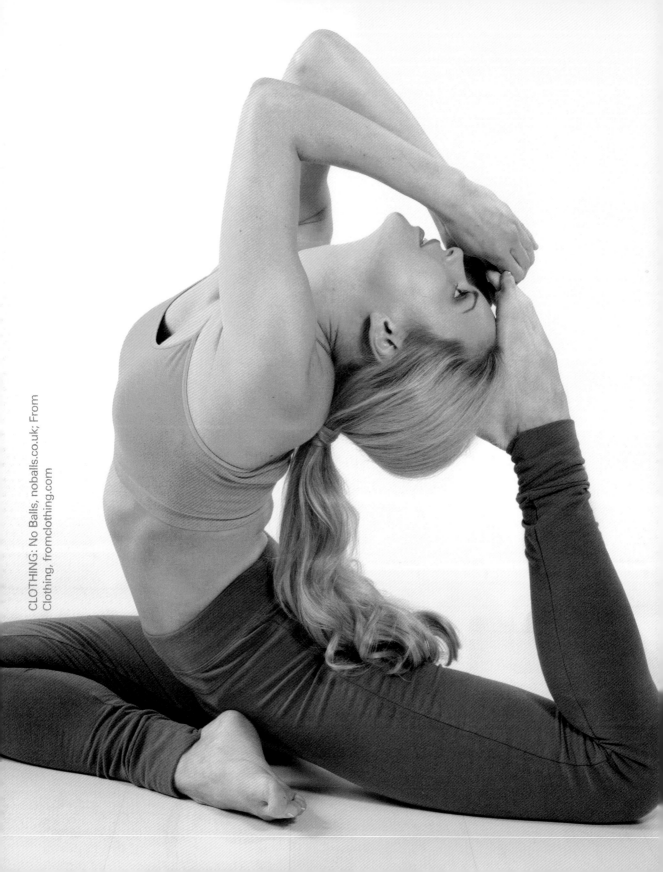

The
SEQUENCES

Now you have the foundations in place, it's time to create a daily practice. This chapter offers yoga sequences for different levels of experience and goals, to suit your needs. Take your time with the sequences. If you need to shorten one, remove postures from the main body of the session. Even if you only practise for 15 minutes, include a warm-up and relaxation for maximum benefit.

Beginner's Sequence

LENGTH: 45 MINUTES

This sequence is designed to safely challenge beginners and give you a grounding in the basic posture categories: standing, balance, sitting, inverted, backbends, supine.

TIP: Hold each posture for four to eight breaths, whatever feels most comfortable – except where otherwise stated. Repeat all the standing and sitting postures to help you get a feel for them. Remember to breathe! If you feel tired, stop, rest and continue focusing on your breath.

1 EASY CROSS-LEGGED POSE
(page 87)
20 breaths

2 WARM-UP SEQUENCE
(page 37)

3 HALF SUN SALUTATIONS
(page 47)
5-7 cycles

4 TRIANGLE
(page 57)

5 WARRIOR II
(page 64)

6 EXTENDED SIDE ANGLE STRETCH WITH ELBOW TO KNEE
(page 66)

7 TREE WITH HANDS IN PRAYER
(page 56)

8 HERO
(page 78)
20 breaths

9 COBBLER
(page 80)

10 ONE LEG BENT SITTING EXTENSION
(page 84)

11 BRIDGE
(page 93)

12 EXTENDED CHILD'S POSE
(page 79)

13 MERMAID
(page 97)

14 BOAT WITH KNEES BENT
(page 88)
Repeat x 3

15 LEGS UP THE WALL
(page 77)
At least 20 breaths

16 CORPSE
(page 103)

3 *Half sun salutations* page 47

2 *Warm-up sequence* page 37

Start

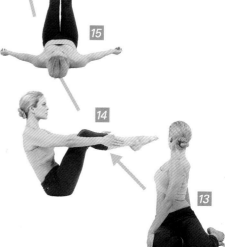

CLOTHING: Wellicious, wellicious.com

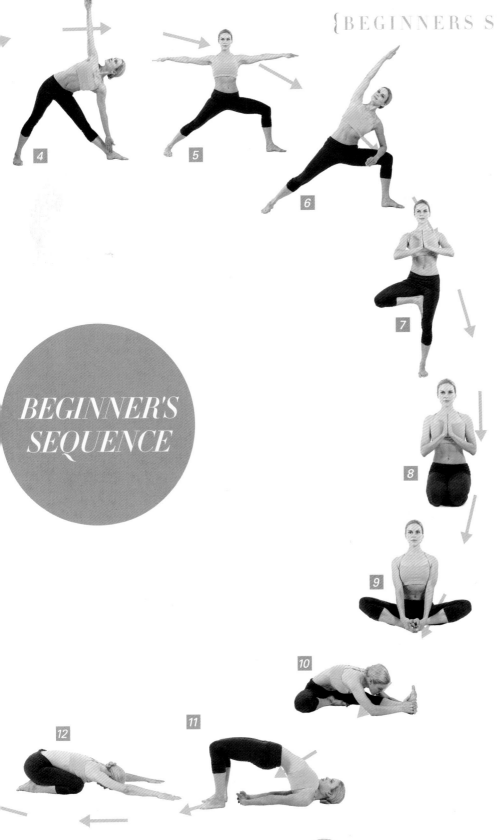

BEGINNER'S SEQUENCE

4

5

6

7

8

9

10

11

12

Times of sequences are approximates, see your doctor before beginning any new exercise routine

Intermediate Sequence - Part I

LENGTH: 60 MINUTES

The emphasis of this sequence is strengthening, opening and relaxing your body through a series of gently challenging poses. Take five to 10 breaths in each pose unless otherwise stated.

TIP: If you feel a pain instead of a deep stretch, stop and breathe, and release your hold on the posture. Remember to practise ahimsa or non violence toward yourself by not pushing beyond your 'edge'.

1 CHILD'S POSE
(page 79)
20 breaths

2 WARM-UP SEQUENCE
(page 37)

3 SUN SALUTATION A
(page 48)
3 rounds

4 SUN SALUTATION B
(page 50)
3 rounds

5 EXTENDED MOUNTAIN
POSE WITH SIDE STRETCH
(page 53)

6 STANDING FORWARD
BEND WITH
DYNAMIC TWIST
(page 60)
5 on each side

7 TREE WITH
ARMS RAISED
(page 56)

8 CHAIR
(page 55)
Repeat x 3

9 DOWNWARD-FACING
DOG
(Page 72)

10 HIGH LUNGE
(page 61)

11 CRESCENT
MOON POSE
(page 62)

12 WARRIOR I
(page 63)

13 WARRIOR III
(page 65)

14 REVOLVED SIDE
ANGLE STRETCH
(page 67)

15 TRIANGLE
(page 57)

Turn to page 110 for Part II of the Intermediate Sequence

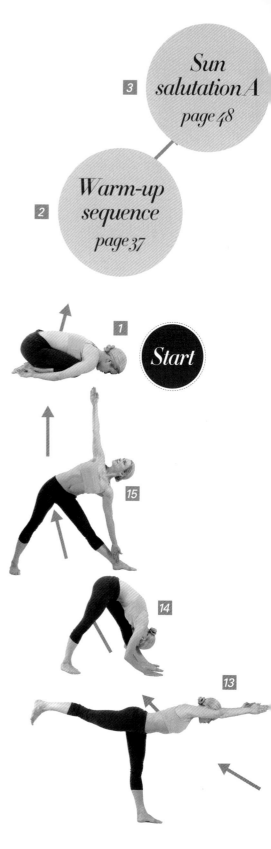

3 *Sun salutation A page 48*

2 *Warm-up sequence page 37*

1 Start

15

14

13

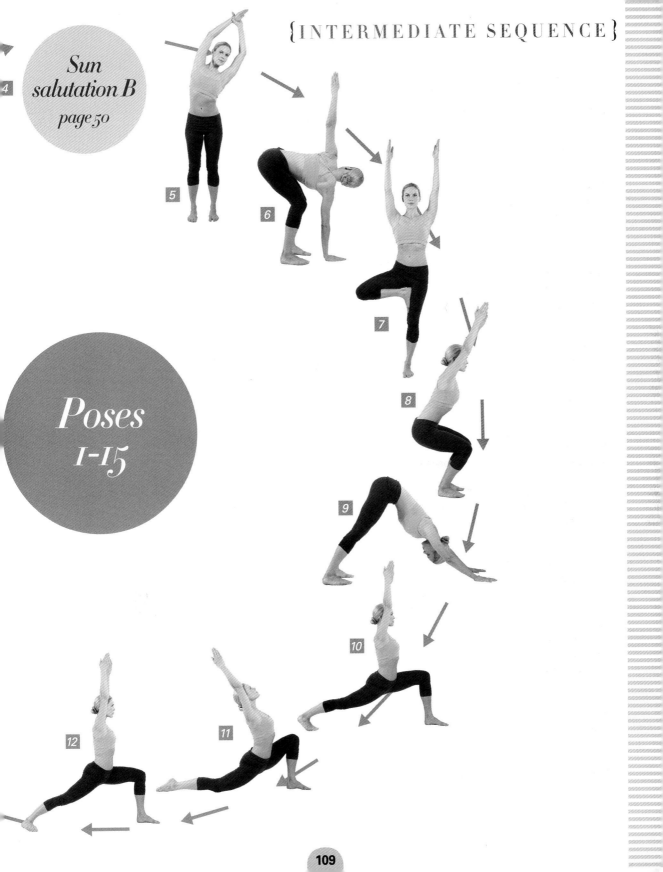

Sun
salutation B
page 50

4

5

6

7

8

9

10

Poses
1-15

11

12

Intermediate Sequence - Part II

CONTINUED FROM PAGE 109

16 REVERSE
TRIANGLE
(page 58)

17 CHILD'S POSE
(page 79)

18 DOWNWARD–FACING
DOG
(page 72)

19 PIGEON WITH
FORWARD BEND
(page 94)

20 SITTING FORWARD
BEND
(page 83)
20 breaths

21 COBBLER
(page 80)

22 CAMEL
(page 92)
Repeat x 2

23 EXTENDED
CHILD'S POSE
(page 79)
20 breaths

24 STANDING FORWARD
BEND DYNAMIC TWIST
(page 60)

25 BOAT
(page 88)
Repeat x 5

26 SHOULDER STAND
(page 74)
10-20 breaths

27 PLOUGH
(page 75)
10-20 breaths

28 KNEES TO CHEST
(rock side to side)
(page 102)

29 STRAIGHT-LEGGED
LYING DOWN TWIST
(page 99)

30 CORPSE
(page 103)
5 minutes

Optional

ALTERNATE NOSTRIL
BREATHING
(page 33)
5 minutes

MINDFUL MEDITATION
(page 35)
5-20 minutes

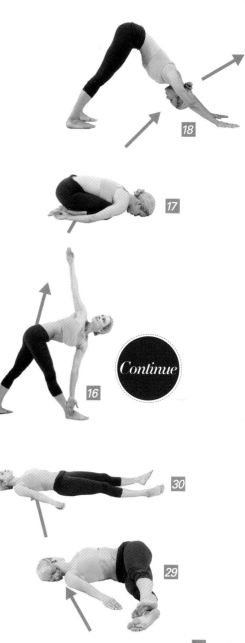

Continue

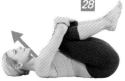

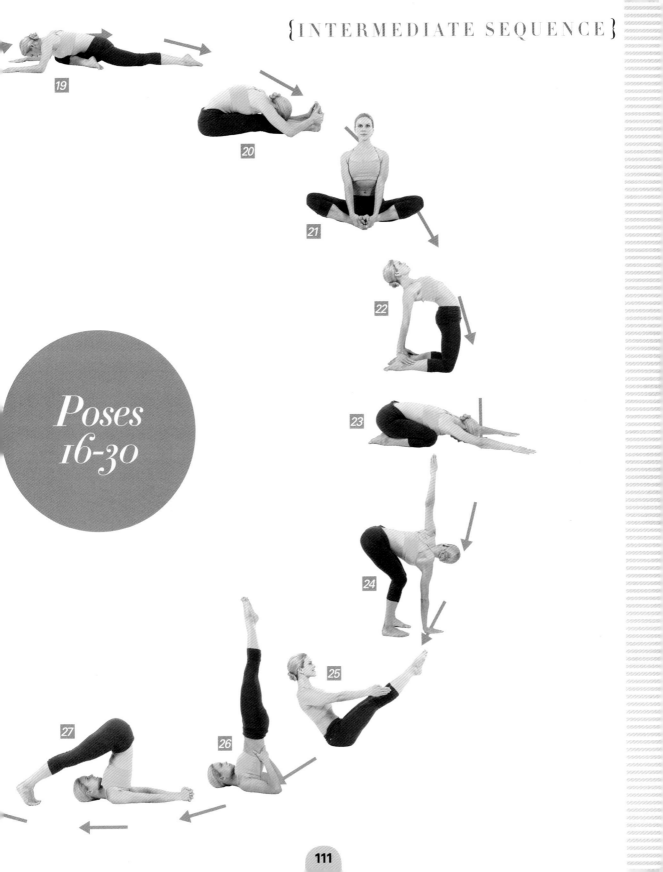

Poses
16-30

Advanced Sequence - Part I

LENGTH: 60-90 MINUTES

A challenging sequence for experienced practitioners or those working through the stages. If you have practised the beginner's and intermediate sequences regularly – at least three times a week – for six weeks each, you may feel ready to move on to this sequence. Remember, use the variations and rest if you're tired!

TIP: Take 10 breaths in each pose unless otherwise stated. Holding the postures for longer enables you to focus more, and absorb the benefits from each pose.

TIP: If you'd like a longer practice, there are repeat options for some postures. If you prefer a shorter session, don't repeat. Never miss your warm-up or final relaxation.

1 CHILD'S POSE
(page 79)
20 breaths

2 WARM-UP SEQUENCE
(pages 37)

3 SUN SALUTATION A
(page 48)
5 cycles

4 SUN SALUTATION B
(page 50)
5 cycles

5 STANDING
FORWARD BEND
(page 54)

6 TRIANGLE
(page 57)
Repeat once

7 REVERSE TRIANGLE
(page 58)

8 WARRIOR II
(page 64)
Repeat once

9 WIDE-LEGGED
FORWARD BEND
(page 68)
Repeat once

10 EXTENDED SIDE
ANGLE POSE
(page 66)
Repeat once

11 WARRIOR I
(page 63)

12 WARRIOR III
(page 65)

13 REVOLVED SIDE
STRETCH
(page 67)
Repeat once

14 DOWNWARD-FACING
DOG
(page 72)

15 DOWNWARD-FACING
DOG SPLITS (PICTURED)
WITH HEAD-TO-KNEE
(page 73)
10 each side

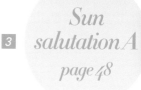

3 *Sun salutation A*
page 48

2 *Warm-up sequence*
page 37

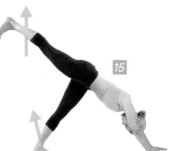

Start

15

14

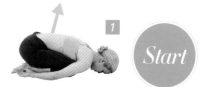

Turn to page 114 for Part II

13

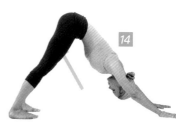

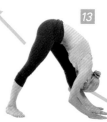

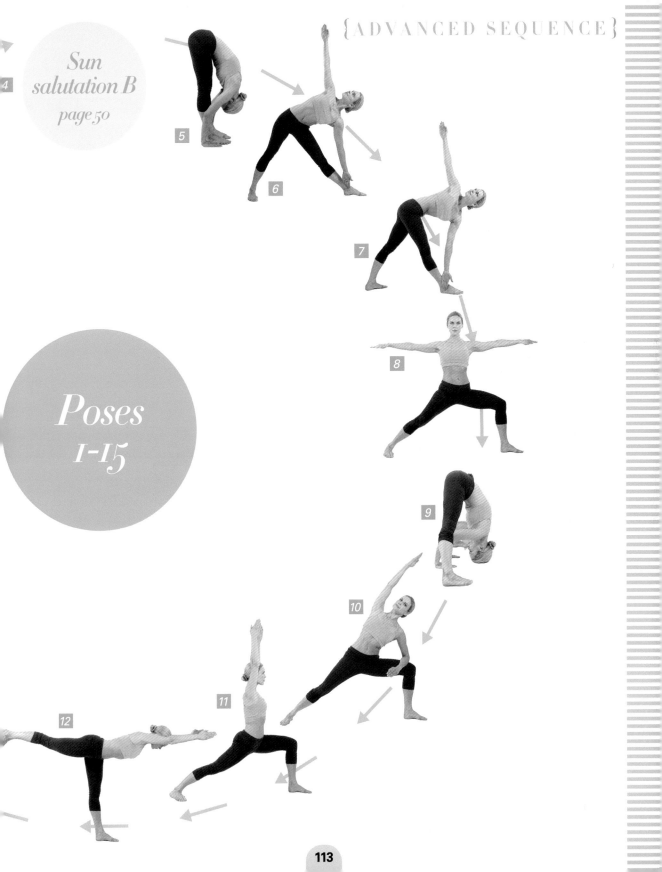

**Sun
salutation B**
page 50

4

5

6

7

8

9

10

11

12

**Poses
1-15**

Advanced
Sequence - Part II

CONTINUED FROM PAGE 113

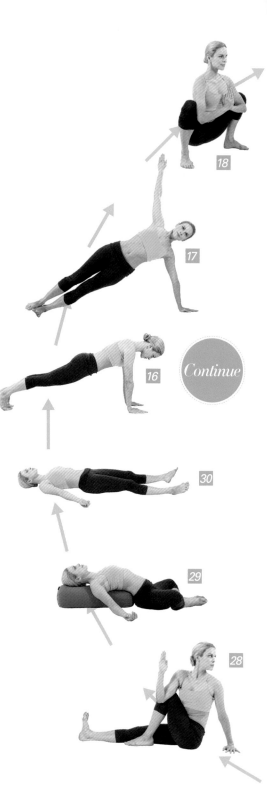

16 PLANK
(page 69)
Repeat x 3

17 SIDE PLANK
(page 70)

18 SQUAT
(page 71)

19 WIDE-LEGGED
FORWARD BEND
(page 68)

20 SITTING
FORWARD BEND
(page 83)

21 DOWNWARD-FACING
DOG
(page 72)

22 HEADSTAND
(page 74)
15-20 breaths

23 CHILD'S POSE
(page 79)
20 breaths

24 BOAT
(page 88)
Repeat x 5

25 COBRA
(page 89)
Repeat x 5

26 WHEEL
(page 95)
Repeat x 2

27 KNEES TO CHEST
(page 102)

28 SEATED SPINE TWIST
(page 98)

29 RECLINING SUPPORTED
COBBLER
(page 81)
20 breaths

30 CORPSE
(page 103)

Optional

BELLOWS BREATH
5 cycles of 15-20 breaths

MINDFULNESS
MEDITATION
5-20 minutes

Continue

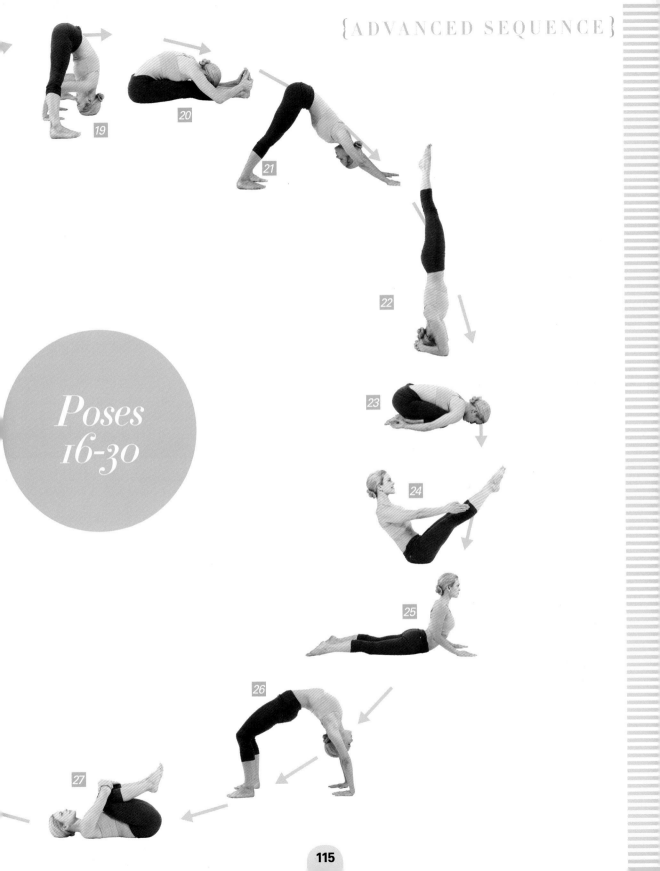

19

20

21

22

23

24

25

26

27

Poses
16-30

Energising Sequence

LENGTH: 30-45 MINUTES

This sequence is designed for anyone feeling sluggish who needs a lift. It's great for morning workouts before work or at lunchtime, and the emphasis is on standing postures and backbends, which enhance energy and lift your mood.

TIP: This sequence can be done posture by posture by coming back to the top of your mat between each pose. Alternatively, flow from one pose to the next.

TIP: Initially, hold each pose for at least five breaths unless otherwise stated. But once familiar with the poses, learn to listen to your body, it knows best.

1 CORPSE
(page 103)
10 breaths

2 WARM UP SEQUENCE
(Pages 37)

3 HALF SUN SALUTATION
(page 47)
5 cycles

4 SUN SALUTATION A
(page 48
5 cycles

5 EXTENDED MOUNTAIN
(page 53)
Repeat 4-5 together x 3

6 CHAIR
(page 55)
Repeat 5-6 together x 3

7 DOWNWARD-FACING DOG
(page 72)

8 DOWNWARD-FACING DOG HEAD-TO-KNEE
(page 54)
5 on each side

9 CHILD'S POSE
(page 79)
20 breaths

10 HIGH LUNGE
(page 61)

11 TRIANGLE
(page 57)

12 HALF MOON POSE
(page 59)

13 COBRA
(page 89)
Repeat x 4

14 LOCUST
(page 90)
Repeat x 4

15 CROSS-LEGGED TWIST
(page 96)
Repeat x 3

16 HAPPY BABY
(page 100)
10-20 breaths

17 CORPSE
(page 103)
5-10 minutes

OPTIONAL

BELLOWS BREATH
3-5 sets of 20 breaths

MINDFUL MEDITATION
2-15 minutes

Half sun salutation
page 47

Warm-up sequence
page 37

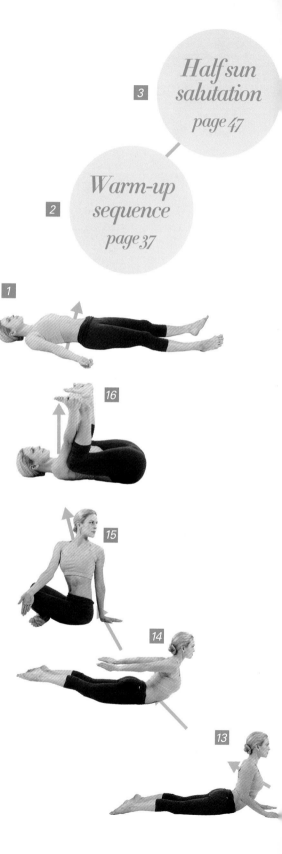

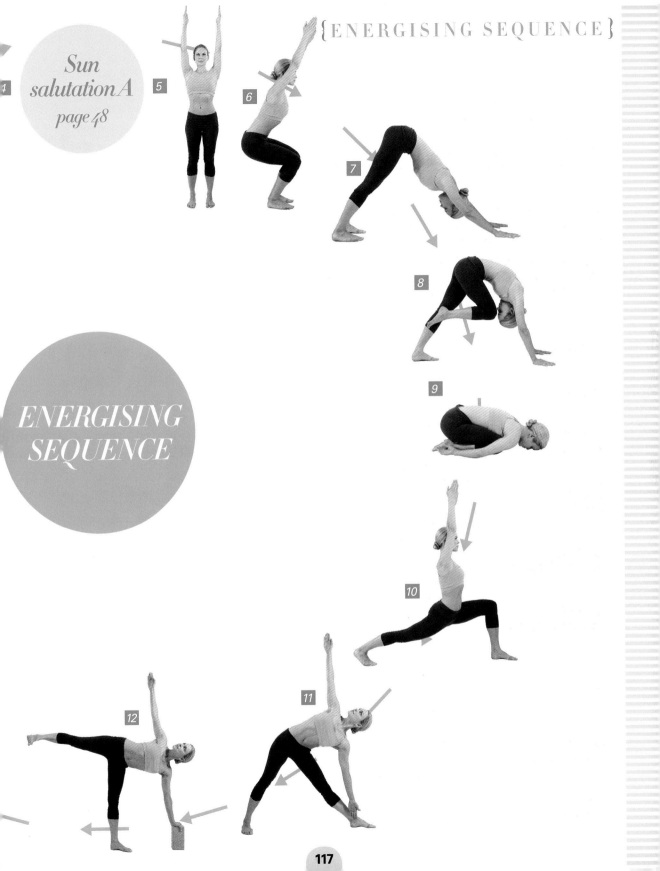

1

Sun salutation A
page 48

5

6

7

ENERGISING SEQUENCE

8

9

10

11

12

Chill-out Sequence

LENGTH: 25-35 MINUTES

This sequence is designed to calm you so is great after work or before bed. The relaxing forward bend postures will draw you into your centre and calm your nervous system. Hold the postures for at least 10 breaths, or if time allows you can take 20 or more long, slow breaths and focus on your breathing becoming longer.

TIP: Hold the final pose, legs up the wall for at least five minutes and, as you come down, rest on the floor on your side before finishing.

1 KNEES TO CHEST
(ROCK SIDE TO SIDE)
(page 102)

2 WARM-UP SEQUENCE
(page 37)

3 EASY CROSS-
LEGGED POSE
(page 87)

4 EASY CROSS-
LEGGED TWIST
(page 96)

5 SEATED CROSS-
LEGGED POSE WITH
FORWARD BEND
(page 87)

6 HERO
(page 78)

7 DOWNWARD-FACING
DOG
(page 72)

8 STANDING FORWARD
BEND KNEES BENT, ARMS
FOLDED, HEAD HANGING
(page 54)

9 MOUNTAIN
(page 52)

10 EXTENDED MOUNTAIN
(page 53)

11 TREE WITH HANDS
IN PRAYER
(page 56)

12 WIDE-LEGGED
FORWARD BEND
(page 68)

13 CHILD'S POSE
(page 79)

14 SITTING
FORWARD BEND
(page 83)

15 COBBLER WITH HEAD
COMING FORWARD
ROUNDED BACK
(Page 81)

16 RECLINING SUPPORTED
COBBLER
(page 81)

17 LEGS UP THE WALL
(AS RELAXATION)
(page 77)
3-10 minutes

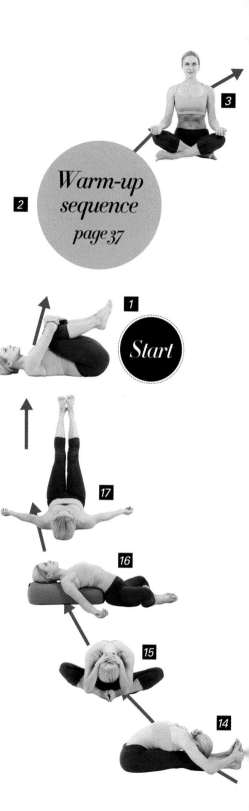

Warm-up sequence page 37

Start

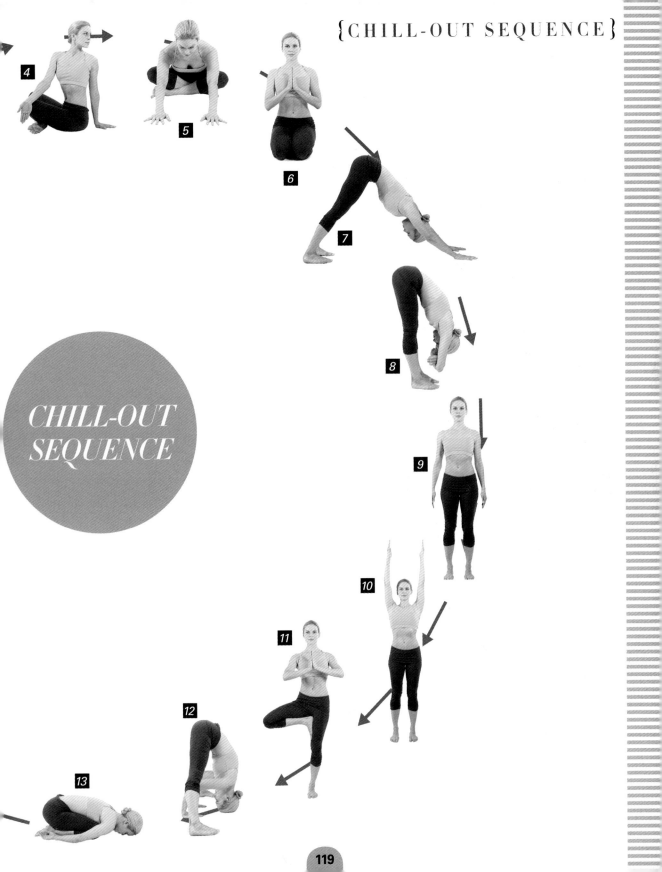

CHILL-OUT
SEQUENCE

4

5

6

7

8

9

10

11

12

13

119

Fat-burning Sequence - Part I

LENGTH: 60 MINUTES

A challenging sequence designed to get your body temperature up and deeply stretch and tone.

TIP: A number of postures in this sequence are repeated to maintain a high body temperature. Always rest in Child's pose if you get tired, and resume when you're ready. Take five to eight breaths in each pose unless otherwise stated.

1 EASY CROSS-LEGGED POSE
(page 87)
20 breaths

2 WARM-UP SEQUENCE
(page 37)

3 SUN SALUTATION A
(page 48)
Three cycles

4 SUN SALUTATION B
(page 50)
Three cycles

5 CHAIR
(page 55)
Repeat x 3

6 STANDING FORWARD BEND
(page 54)

7 DOWNWARD-FACING DOG
(page 72)

8 PLANK
(page 69)
Repeat x 3

9 SIDE PLANK
(page 70)

10 WARRIOR I
(page 63)

11 WARRIOR II
(page 64)

12 EXTENDED SIDE ANGLE POSE
(page 66)

13 TRIANGLE
(page 57)

14 REVERSE TRIANGLE
(page 58)

15 STANDING WIDE-LEGGED FORWARD BEND
(page 68)

Turn to page 122 for Part II

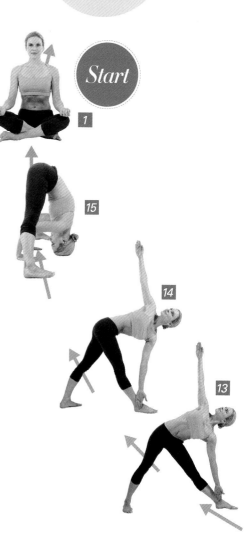

3 *Sun salutation A page 48*

2 *Warm-up sequence page 37*

Start

1

15

14

13

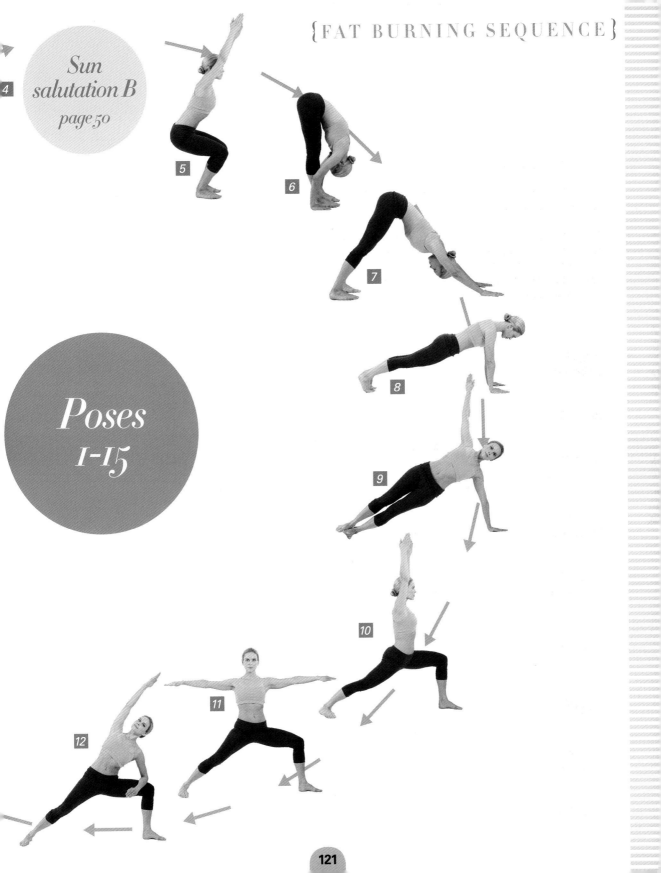

Sun
salutation B
page 50

4

5

6

7

8

9

Poses
1-15

10

11

12

Fat-burning Sequence - Part II

CONTINUED FROM PAGE 121

16 TREE WITH HANDS IN PRAYER
(page 56)

17 SQUAT
(page 71)

18 COBRA
(page 89)

19 LOCUST
(page 90)

20 BOW
(page 91)
repeat x 3

21 EXTENDED CHILD'S POSE
(page 79)

22 SITTING FORWARD BEND
(page 83)

23 SEATED SPINE TWIST
(page 98)

24 COBBLER
(page 80)

25 BRIDGE
(page 93)
Repeat x 3

26 SHOULDER STAND
(page 74)
20 breaths

27 HAPPY BABY
(page 100)

28 BOAT
(Page 88)
Repeat x 5

29 EASY CROSS-LEGGED POSE FORWARD BEND
(page 87)
20 breaths

30 CORPSE
(page 103)
10 minutes

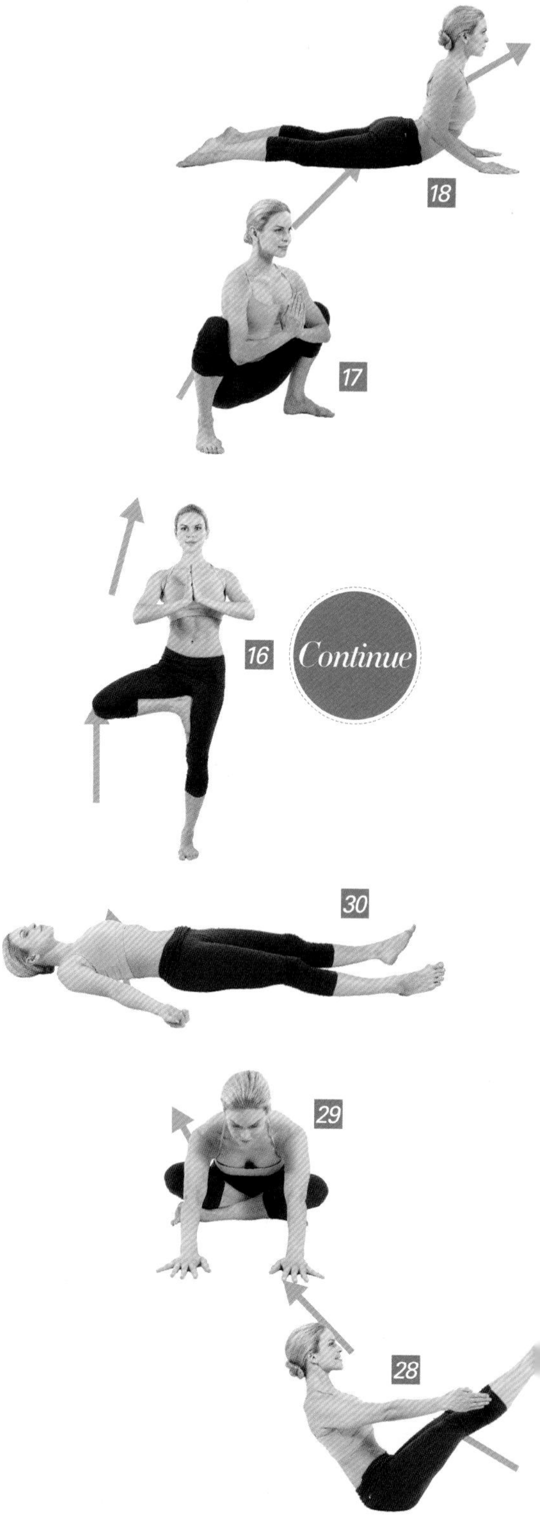

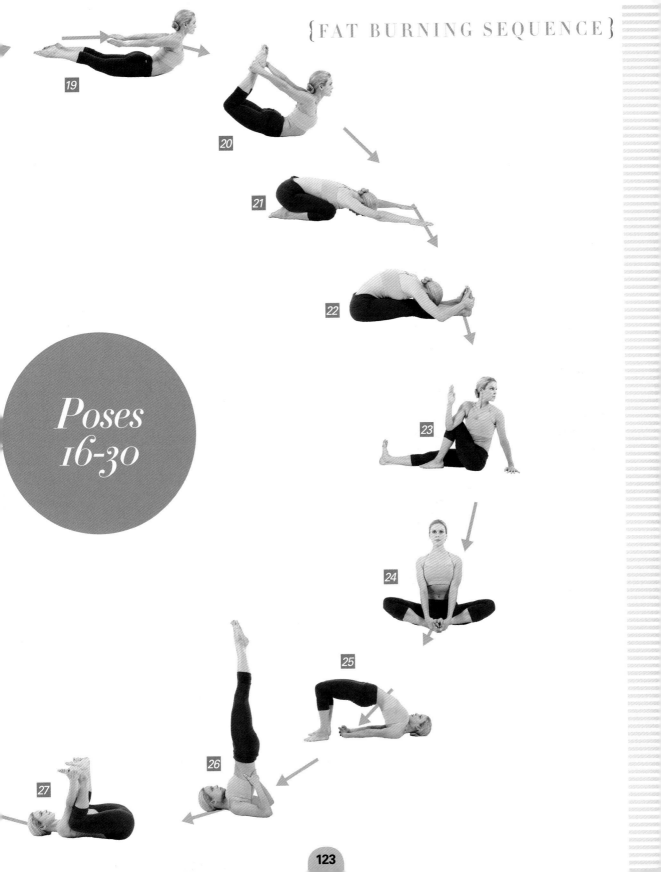

19

20

21

22

Poses
16-30

23

24

25

26

27

Six-week plan for
BEGINNERS

You're now ready to start a daily yoga practice that will calm and energise, tone your body and increase your flexibility

*I*f you're just starting out, take your practice slowly so that you can experience the benefits of yoga for yourself – safely and without injury. This six-week course has been designed to help you gradually build up your practice to intermediate level. It's based on four practice days a week that you can do anytime.

After the first six weeks, continue to practise by alternating the beginner's and intermediate sequences for the next eight to 12 weeks, until you feel ready to move on to a more advanced practice. Remember to look for a good teacher who can ensure you are not developing unsafe habits.

Enjoy!

	WEEK 1	WEEK 2	WEEK 3	WEEK 4	WEEK 5	WEEK 6
DAY 1	Warm-up Sequence (page 37)	Warm-up Sequence Half sun salutation x 5 Sun salutation A (page 48) x 3	Chill-out Sequence (page 118)	Beginner's Sequence	Warm-up Sequence Sun salutation A x 3 Sun salutation B x 3 (page 50)	Beginner's Sequence
DAY 2	Half sun salutation x 5	Beginner's Sequence (page 106)	Beginner's Sequence	Beginner's Sequence	Intermediate Sequence (page 108)	Intermediate Sequence
DAY 3	Warm-up Sequence Half sun salutation x 5	Warm-up Sequence Half sun salutation x 5 Sun salutation A x 3	Warm-up Sequence Half sun salutation x 5 Sun salutation A x 3	Beginner's Sequence	Warm-up Sequence Sun salutation A x 3 Sun salutation B x 3	Beginner's Sequence
DAY 4	Warm-up Sequence Half sun salutation x 5 Sun salutation A x 3	Beginner's Sequence	Beginner's Sequence	Chill-out Sequence	Intermediate Sequence	Intermediate sequence

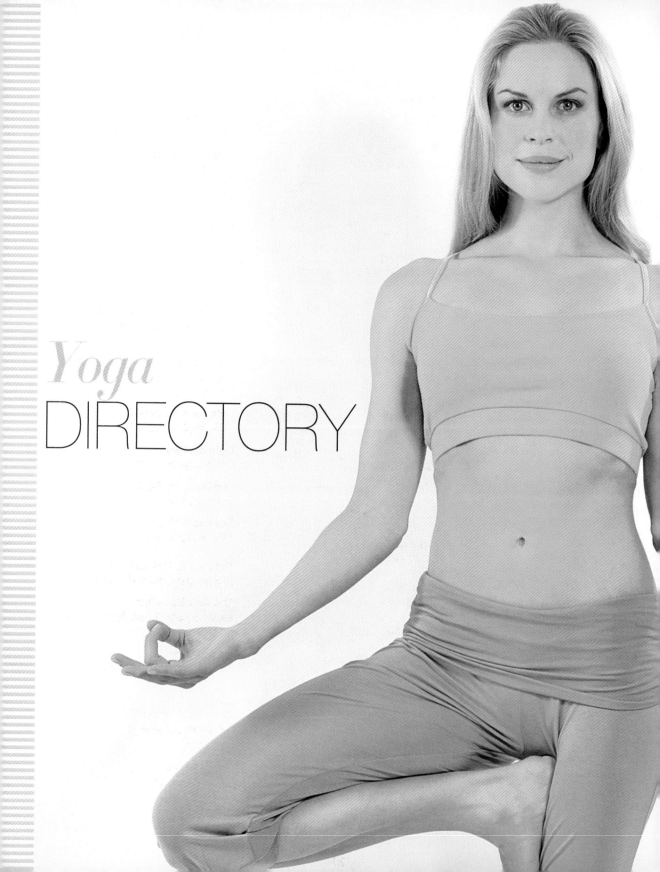

Yoga
DIRECTORY

Apparel

Casall
casall.co.uk
01458 274557

Freddy
freddy.com

From Clothing
fromclothing.com
01404 510518

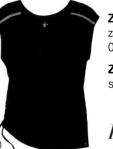
Moving Comfort

Let your body breathe
letyourbodybreathe.com
020 7193 6342

Lululemon
lululemon.co.uk

Manuka
manukalife.com

Moving Comfort
movingcomfort.com

No Balls
noballs.co.uk
01638 570387

Panache
panache-lingerie.com

No Balls

Sheactive
sheactive.co.uk
0845 094 9434

Striders Edge
stridersedge.co.uk

Sweaty Betty
sweatybetty.co.uk

USA Pro
sportsdirect.com

Urban Yoga
urbanyoga.co.uk
0845 519 7121

Wellicious
wellicious.com

Yoga Matters
yogamatters.com
020 8888 8588

Yoga Matters

Zaggora
zaggora.com
07537 404575

Zoca
sheactive.co.uk/zoca

Food and supplements

Good Hemp
goodwebsite.co.uk

Maxitone
maxitone.com
01442 244330

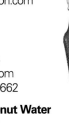
Good Hemp

Reflex
reflex-nutrition.com

Solgar
solgar.com

Vitabiotics
vitabiotics.com
020 8955 2662

ZICO Coconut Water
uk.zico.com

Zico

Yoga centres and classes

Astanga Yoga
astangayogalondon.com

Triyoga
triyoga.co.uk

Wellington Centre
thewellingtoncentre.com

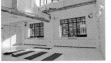
Triyoga

Yoga Place
yogaplace.co.uk

Websites

Glowgetter.co.uk
General merchandise and information

Myyogaonline.com
Video classes

Yogaglo.com
Video classes

Yogamatters.com
Props and books

Books

Asana Pranayama Mudra Bandha
Swami Satyananda Saraswati
(Yoga Publications Trust)

Ashtanga Yoga: The Practice Manual
David Swenson
(Are You Practising)

Light on Pranayama
BKS Iyengar (Crossroad)

Light on Yoga
BKS Iyengar (Harper Collins)

The Breathing Book
Donna Farhi (Holt)

The Heart of Yoga
TKV Desikachar (Inner Traditions)

The Path To Holistic Health
BKS Iyengar (Dorling Kindersley)

The Yoga Body Diet
Kristen Schultz Dollard, John Douillard
(Rodale)

Yoga for You
Tara Fraser (Duncan Baird Publications)

Find a teacher

British Wheel of Yoga
bwy.org.uk

Yoga Alliance
yogaalliance.co.uk

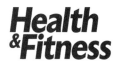
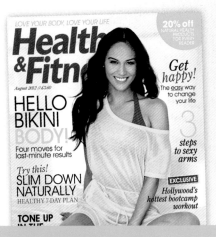

e hope that you've enjoyed discovering the many incredible benefits of yoga while working through this book. Whether you've followed the sessions and six-week plan religiously, or simply dipped in and out to try new poses, hopefully you're now feeling toned and healthy, as well as a little more bendy! Keeping up a regular yoga practice is one of the very best things you can do for your health and wellbeing. We hope this is just the start of your yoga journey.